Second Edition

Acne

Atlas with Treatment Options

Second Edition

Acne

Atlas with Treatment Options

Bela J Shah
Professor and Head
Department of Dermatology Venereology and Leprology
BJ Medical College and Civil Hospital
Ahmedabad, Gujarat

CBSPD

CBS Publishers & Distributors Pvt Ltd

New Delhi • Bengaluru • Chennai • Kochi • Kolkata • Lucknow • Mumbai
Gujarat • Hyderabad • Jharkhand • Nagpur • Patna • Pune • Uttarakhand

Disclaimer

Science and technology are constantly changing fields. New research and experience broaden the scope of information and knowledge. The author has tried her best in giving information available to her while preparing the material for this book. Although all efforts have been made to ensure optimum accuracy of the material, yet it is quite possible some errors might have been left uncorrected. The publisher, the printer and the author will not be held responsible for any inadvertent errors, omissions or inaccuracies.

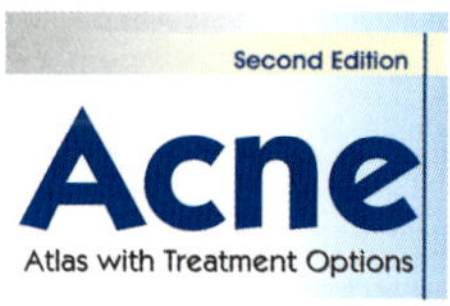

ISBN: 978-93-5466-804-3

Second Edition: 2026

First Edition: 2018

Published by Satish Kumar Jain and produced by Varun Jain for

CBS Publishers & Distributors Pvt Ltd

4819/XI Prahlad Street, 24 Ansari Road, Daryaganj, New Delhi 110 002, India
Ph: 011-23289259, 23266838 Website: www.cbspd.com
e-mail: delhi@cbspd.com

Corporate Office: 204 FIE, Industrial Area, Patparganj, Delhi 110 092, India
Ph: 011-4934 4934 Fax: 011-4934 4935 e-mail: publishing@cbspd.com; publicity@cbspd.com

Branches

- **Bengaluru:** Seema House 2975, 17th Cross, KR Road, Banasankari 2nd Stage, Bengaluru 560 070, Karnataka, India
  Ph: +91-80-26771678/79 Fax: +91-80-26771680 e-mail: bangalore@cbspd.com
- **Chennai:** 18/8B, Subbarayan Street, Shenoy Nagar, Chennai 600 030, Tamil Nadu, India
  Ph: +91-44-42032115, 26681266 e-mail: chennai@cbspd.com
- **Kochi:** 42/1325, 1326, Power House Road, Opp KSEB, Power House, Ernakulum 682 018, Kochi Kerala, India
  Ph: +91-484-4059061-65,67 Fax: +91-484-4059065 e-mail: kochi@cbspd.com
- **Kolkata:** 147, Hind Ceramics Compound, 1st Floor, Nilgunj Road, Belghoria, Kolkata 700 056, West Bengal, India
  Ph: +033-25633055/56 e-mail: kolkata@cbspd.com
- **Lucknow:** Basement, Khushnuma Complex, 7 Meerabai Marg (behind Jawahar Bhawan), Lucknow 226 001, UP, India
  Ph: +0522-4000032 e-mail: tiwari.lucknow@cbspd.com
- **Mumbai:** PWD Shed, Gala no 25/26, Ramchandra Bhatt Marg, Next to JJ Hospital Gate no. 2, Opp. Union Bank of India, Noorbaug, Mumbai 400 009, Maharashtra, India
  Ph: +022-66661880/89 e-mail: mumbai@cbspd.com

Representatives

- **Gujarat** 0-9879558667
- **Nagpur** 0-8692091830
- **Uttarakhand** 0-9716462459
- **Hyderabad** 0-9885175004
- **Patna** 0-9334159340
- **Jharkhand** 0-9811541605
- **Pune** 0-9664372571

Printed at: Gokul Offset Pvt. Ltd, Okhla Industrial Area, New Delhi, India

Foreword

Government of India
Ministry of Health and Family Welfare
Department of Dermatology, STD and Leprosy
PGIMER and Dr Ram Manohar Lohia Hospital
New Delhi 110001

This book is a sincere attempt to picturize and present concisely a disorder which is arguably the most common skin disorder. The book covers in brief almost all the aspects that encompass the various aspects of the disease with a focus on treatments, both medical and cosmetic. Truly *Acne* encompasses almost all the aspects of clinical practice, though most focus on the cosmetic aspects which might not be needed if it is managed correctly.

The classification, tables and photographs are appropriate and the general practitioners shall find it highly advantageous in their daily medical practice. The postgraduate students will find this compact book a handy addendum in their clinical practice.

It is truly amazing that with a busy and taxing schedule in the largest medical college hospital in Gujarat, encumbered by her multiple assignment, Prof Bela J Shah has managed this book.

I wish the author success in this endeavour.

Dr (Prof) Kabir Sardana
MD, DNB, MNAMS
Professor (Skin & VD), Central Health Services
Professor (Dermatology), Indraprastha University, Delhi
Skin Physician to Dr Ram Manohar Lohia Hospital
Delhi 110001

Preface

It gives me immense pleasure to present this book *Acne Atlas with Treatment Options* in its second edition.

Our understanding of acne has undergone dramatic change over the last couple of years in terms of its epidemiology, pathogenesis, clinical variants, etc. Acne is no longer considered to be a disease of adolescence but can affect anyone from pediatric to geriatric age group. Moreover, many systemic drugs especially. Newer targeted therapies result into acneiform eruptions. Rarely, it can be part of few uncommon syndromes. There is tremendous research and new insights into the current and potential treatment strategies for the management of acne as well as scars.

This book is meant to be a ready-reckoner for busy practising dermatologists, residents, postgraduate students and family physicians alike.

I wish to specially thank my postgraduate resident, Dr Tejasvi Patel, for her hardwork, utmost dedication and untiring efforts at every stage, throughout the compilation of this book.

Finally, I wish to thank CBS Publishers & Distributors for publishing this book.

Bela J Shah

Contents

CHAPTER

1

Background

Acne is a highly prevalent chronic inflammatory disorder of pilosebaceous unit (hair follicle and related sebaceous gland) and presents most commonly as comedones which can be open or closed and inflammatory lesions like papules, pustules, nodules and cysts which can result into post-inflammatory hyperpigmentation and variable degree of disfiguring scars.

It is considered to be most commonly reported condition in dermatological clinic. Acne can have a prolonged course with acute or insidious onset and frequent recurrences. It affects a large percentage of population at some stage of life. It is most common during puberty but also reported as early as 9 years of age as well as in the adult age group. Approximately 85% of people between the age of 12 to 24 experience minor form of acne, e.g. comedones.

When used generally, the term acne refers to acne vulgaris but other variants of acne like monomorphic acne, acne conglobata, acne fulminans, acne excoriée, pomade acne, chloracne and neonatal acne, etc. are well-established entities.

Acne can be found in association with few syndromes. Symptoms suggestive of SAHA (seborrhoea, acne, hirsutism, androgenetic alopecia) syndrome, SAPHO (synovitis, acne, pustulosis, hyperostosis, osteitis) syndrome, PAPA (pyogenic sterile arthritis, pyoderma gangrenosum, acne), Apert syndrome, HAIR-AN (hyperandrogenism, insulin resistance, acanthosis nigricans) have been described in literature. PASH and PAPASH are newly reported syndromes related to acne.

Various mechanisms are proposed for acne pathogenesis like increased sebaceous gland activity with seborrhoea, abnormal follicular differentiation with abnormal keratinisation, microbial colonization of the follicular canal. Role of toll-like receptors and matrix metalloproteinases is now being increasingly recognized in the pathogenesis of acne. Other important contributing factors like diet (high glycemic index food), IGF-1, IL-17, genetic factors, stress, smoking, etc. should be looked at while dealing with the patients of acne.

Nowadays, *Propionibacterium* acnes resistance to conventional (macrolides) antibiotic therapy is widely reported.

In cases of overt cutaneous signs and symptoms of hyperandrogenism, before starting any therapy, thorough investigation in form of hormonal profile should be done and accordingly, therapy should be individualised.

Various modalities of treatment available are antibiotics, hormonal therapy, laser therapy, photodynamic therapy and topical therapy. Lifestyle modification and diet modification are also important steps in the treatment ladder. Various aesthetic procedures such as chemical peels, microdermabrasion, subcision, lasers and light treatments are being utilised for acne, acne scars and pigmentation.

Acne is no longer just a part of growing up process or cosmetic problem but a common cause of anxiety, depression, social phobia, low self-esteem and psychological problems that affect patients' quality of life. The psychological and social impact of acne is a challenge for health care providers because it affects adolescents at crucial stage of life when they are developing their personalities. Early and effective management may promote better healing and reduces the chances of scarring, thus reducing the psychological impact of acne and its sequel.

CHAPTER

2

History

The sixth-century Greek physician Aëtius of Amida is credited with coining the term "ionthos" (ιονθωξ) or "acnae", which is believed to have been a reference to facial skin lesions that occur during "the 'acme' of life" (puberty). The ancient Egyptians used the term aku-t, which means boils, blains, sore, pustules, or any inflamed swelling. Elyot may have seen acne as part of a wider endocrinological syndrome because he describes obesity of the upper body that is associated with boils, increased urine, and black pouches. In the 16th century, the French physician and botanist François Boissier de Sauvages de Lacroix provided one of the earlier descriptions of acne. He used the term "psydracia achne" to describe small, red and hard tubercles that altered a person's facial appearance during adolescence, and were neither itchy nor painful.

In 1638, Riolanus associated acne with menstruation–related disorders. Given its phonetic resemblance to the term we use today, this likely represents the root word of acne. The recognition and characterization of acne progressed in 1776 when Josef Plenck (an Austrian physician) published a book that proposed the novel concept of classifying skin diseases by their elementary (initial) lesions. The term acne vulgaris (vulgaris means common) was first used by Fuchs in 1840 and has persisted to the present day.[1]

Skin glands were identified after the invention of microscopes. Italian researcher Marcello Malpighi discussed pores as the opening of glands in the skin in his book *Opera Postuma*. Hermann Boerhaave, a Dutch Professor of Medicine and Botanics, also supported this view. The term sebaceous gland was coined by Giovanni Battista Morgagni, who described them in his book *De Sedibus et cause morborum per anatomen indagatis.*

In 1808 the English dermatologist Robert Willan refined Plenck's work by providing the first detailed descriptions of several skin disorders using a morphologic terminology that remains in use today. Thomas Bateman continued and expanded on Robert Willan's work as his student and provided the first descriptions and illustrations of acne accepted as accurate by modern dermatologists. English dermatologist, Samuel Plumbe, in 1837 described blockage of the sebaceous glands. In the 19th century, Robert Willan and Thomas Bateman, divided acne into four types based on the associated lesions: Simplex, punctate, indurate, and rosacea.[2]

Erasmus Wilson, in 1842, was the first to make the distinction between acne vulgaris and rosacea. The first professional medical monograph dedicated entirely to acne was published in New York in 1885.

Scientists initially hypothesized that acne represented a disease of the skin's hair follicle, and occurred due to blockage of the pore by sebum. During the 1880s, bacteria were observed by microscopy in skin samples affected by acne and were regarded as the causal agents of comedones, sebum production, and ultimately acne. During the mid-20th century, dermatologists realized that no single hypothesized factor (sebum, bacteria, or excess keratin) could completely explain the disease. This led to the current understanding that acne could be explained by a sequence of related events, beginning with the blockage of the skin follicle by excessive dead skin cells, followed by bacterial invasion of the hair follicle pore, changes in sebum production, and inflammation.

The understanding of the multifactorial pathophysiology of acne vulgaris has considerably improved over the years. There is a genetic component associated with acne vulgaris, hence, it is thought to be familial in half of the cases. Today acne is recognized as an inflammatory process in which *Propionibacterium acnes* and innate immunity trigger a cascade of events at the level of the pilosebaceous unit that break down triglycerides to release free fatty acids, produce substances that are chemotactic for inflammatory cells, and induce the ductal epithelium to secrete pro-inflammatory cytokines (interleukin [IL]-1, IL-6, IL-8, IL-10, IL-12 and tumor necrosis factor-alpha [TNF-α]). The inflammatory reaction continues by means of a type IV immune reaction to one or more antigens in the follicle. Current understanding is that inflammation, namely the expression of IL-α from the open comedones, precedes abnormal hyperkeratinization.

TREATMENT THROUGH THE AGES

While Greeks preferred vegetable-based treatments for acne, Egyptians typically opted for animal-based products. The most common treatment they used was honey. Pharaohs are recorded as having had acne, which may be the earliest known reference to the disease. Since at least the reign of Cleopatra (69–30 BC), the application of sulfur to the skin has been recognized as a useful treatment for acne.

Throughout the Middle Ages, the four humors that underpinned medical treatment and research was stifled by religious control. Treatment development stagnated and was based on balancing humors, diets, herbal remedies, and prayers.

Botanical and herbal treatments were still used till 1936. Goodman first stated the importance of a good history that includes information about diet, cathartics, periods, urine, blood sugar, ingestion of bromide or iodine drugs, blood purifiers, headache medicine, nerve tonics, and sleep potions. Topical treatments were classified into keratolytic, antiseptic, astringent, emollient, and keratoplastic therapies.

1% hydrocortisone, a mid-1900s medication was claimed to cure acne.

Goodman discussed peels and recommended an initial application for 1 to 3 hours and, if the patient had no adverse reaction, to extend the peel for a full treatment lasting 12 hours. The peels he described contained (a) 40 parts resorcin, 10 parts zinc oxide, 6 parts kaolin, 100 parts benzoinate lard, and (b) 32 parts resorcin, 20 parts potash soap, 20 parts sulfur lotum, and 100 parts spirits of lavender. Antiseptic therapies as recommended by Goodman were iodine, picric acid, sodium carbonate, camphor, alcohol, and boric or oleic acids.

Canadian dermatologist William E Pace was the first to recognize the usefulness of benzoyl peroxide to treat acne. MacKee and his team advised in 1922 that "avoiding candy, pastry, soda water, ice cream, chocolate, rich foods, fried foods, cocoa and gravy as a bare minimum plus or minus tea, coffee, alcohol and spices". Goodman praised the following foods as suitable to cure acne: Cooked and raw fruit, farina, rice, wheat, oatmeal, green vegetables, boiled or broiled meat and poultry, clear soup, vegetable soup, and an abundance of water.

The approach to acne treatment underwent significant changes during the 20th century.

In the first half of the 20th century, phototherapy was a popular treatment for acne and quartz mercury vapor lamps in particular were used.

Retinoids were introduced as a medical treatment for acne in 1943. Benzoyl peroxide was first proposed as a treatment in 1958 and has been routinely used for this purpose since 1960s. Acne treatment was modified in 1950s with the introduction of oral tetracycline antibiotics (such as minocycline).

These reinforced the idea amongst dermatologists that bacterial growth on the skin plays an important role in causing acne. Subsequently, in 1970s tretinoin (original trade name Retin A) was found to be an effective treatment.

The development of oral isotretinoin (sold as Accutane and Roaccutane) followed in 1980.

Oral zinc has been used extensively both topically and systemically for the management of acne vulgaris ever since the time its favorable effect on acne was recognized by Michaelsson in a patient of acrodermatitis enteropathica and subsequent studies demonstrated low serum zinc in acne patient. Oral zinc sulfate is reportedly more effective in the treatment of severe acne than for the treatment of mild to moderate acne. Recently, a methionine bound zinc complex with antioxidants has been tried and found useful in managing mild to moderate acne vulgaris zinc, with or without nicotinamide, is also another emerging alternate acne treatment to reduce adverse effect of antibiotics.

In Japan and a few European countries, nadifloxacin has been approved for the treatment of acne vulgaris.

Orally dapsone has been used in the past for recalcitrant acne (in the doses of 25–50 mg/day) but haematological and other complications limit its use.

A topical gel formulation of Dapsone 5% was developed and approved by The United States Food and Drug Administration (USFDA) in 2005.

REFERENCES

1. Grant RNR. The History of Acne. Proceedings of the Royal Society of Medicine. 1951;44(8):647–52.
2. Mahmooda NF, Shipmana AR. The age-old problem of acne. Int J Womens Dermatol. 2017 Jun; 3(2): 71–6.

CHAPTER

3

Epidemiology

Acne vulgaris affects approximately 40–50 million individuals each year in the US alone.

We do not have exact Indian data. All races worldwide suffer from this disease and it affects more than 90% of people at sometime or the other in their lives.

In India, prevalence data from a dermatology clinic in a teaching hospital in Varanasi reported acne in 50.6% of boys and 38.13% of girls in the age group of 12–17 years. There are believed to be no gender differences in acne prevalence, although such differences are often reported and, very likely, represent social biases. In clinics in the urban areas, there is a clear preponderance of girls seeking treatment but that scene is fast changing. There is also a perception that acne is less prevalent in rural population. This is supported by the data from Varanasi where 21.35% of boys (13–18 years) from rural areas had acne versus 37.5% from the urban areas.

Actually this may not be the case nowadays.

AGE AND GENDER

Acne affects approximately 85% of young people between 12 and 24 years of age, showing a peak incidence during adolescence. Hence, it is considered a physiological occurrence in this group. The age of onset is at puberty or a few months earlier. The peak incidence is between 14 and 17 years in women and 16–19 years in men. Typically considered a disease of youth, acne often continues to be problematic even into adulthood.

It was earlier regarded as a transient disease of the teenage years, however, acne is now seen presenting earlier and lasting longer. This earlier development of acne is likely due to earlier onset of puberty, which is also linked to diet/obesity and other lifestyle factors. Girls develop acne at a younger age than boys due to earlier adrenarche.[1–3] Neonatal acne resulting from circulating maternal hormones is also known to occur.

Before any overt signs of puberty, some children may show comedonal acne. This is linked with the pathophysiology of acne where increased adrenal dihydroepiandrosterone (DHEA-S) output results in sebum production in androgen susceptible follicles in both girls and boys. Early adrenarche in girls is a known risk factor for polycystic ovary syndrome (PCOS), metabolic syndrome and insulin resistance.[4] Girls showing early development of comedonal acne may suffer from more severe disease even later in life.

Males suffer from acne more commonly than females and the severity of acne is also more, which is related to androgen activity. There are very few epidemiological studies from India, but two studies from north and one from south confirmed male preponderance and urban population being affected more than rural. Premenstrual flare in majority of females was also reported in the study from south. A more severe grade of acne vulgaris was seen in smokers compared to non-smokers.

Post-adolescent acne, both persistent and late onset, is seen to be much more common in women than in men.[3, 5, 6] A number of studies, both old and recent, have reported that males have more severe acne in late adolescence than girls.[1, 7–9] The age distribution of acne is widening in both sexes but more prominently in women over the age of 40 years.

Endocrine disorders such as hypercortisolism, precocious puberty, polycystic ovarian syndrome and hyperandrogenism are associated with more severe acne that is less responsive to standard therapy.

RACE AND ETHNICITY

A few racial differences are known. The American population is said to be affected more than the Japanese. Caucasian boys and men show a predisposition for more severe nodulocystic disease than other groups. Peak prevalence occurs between the ages of

15 and 20 years in all ethnic groups. It is extremely challenging to unravel the effects of ethnicity, socioeconomic and cultural factors as has been shown by epidemiological studies. However, ethnic variation in the prevalence of acne is shown to exist even when socioeconomic and cultural factors are accounted for.

GENETICS

The susceptibility to acne is influenced by genetic factors. Children having acne especially severe grades have one or both parents having acne in many cases. The similarity of lesions in monozygotic twins and racial predisposition has also been considered to exist due to genetic factors. An XYY karyotype individual carries an increased risk for the development of acne.[10]

REFERENCES

1. Stathakis V, Kilkenny M, Marks R. Descriptive epidemiology of acne vulgaris in the community. Australasian Journal of Dermatology. 1997;38(3):115–23.
2. Wu TQ, Mei SQ, Zhang JX, Gong LF, Wu FJ, Wu WH, Li J, Lin M, Diao JX. Prevalence and risk factors of facial acne vulgaris among Chinese adolescents. International Journal of Adolescent Medicine and Health. 2007 Oct;19(4):407–12.
3. Shen Y, Wang T, Zhou C, Wang X, Ding X, Tian S, Liu Y, Peng G, Xue S, Zhou J, Wang R. Prevalence of acne vulgaris in Chinese adolescents and adults: a community-based study of 17,345 subjects in six cities. Acta Dermato-venereologica. 2012;92(1):40–4.
4. Ibáñez L, DiMartino-Nardi J, Potau N, Saenger P. Premature adrenarche—normal variant or forerunner of adult disease?. Endocrine Reviews. 2000 Dec 1;21(6):671–96.
5. Goulden, Mcgeown, Cunliffe. The familial risk of adult acne: a comparison between first-degree relatives of affected and unaffected individuals. British Journal of Dermatology. 1999 Aug;141(2):297–300.
6. Khunger N, Kumar C. A clinico-epidemiological study of adult acne: is it different from adolescent acne?. Indian Journal of Dermatology, Venereology and Leprology. 2012 May 1;78:335.
7. Rombouts S, Nijsten T, Lambert J. Cigarette smoking and acne in adolescents: results from a cross-sectional study. Journal of the European Academy of Dermatology and Venereology. 2007 Mar;21(3):326–33.

8. Hanisah A, Omar K, Shah SA. Prevalence of acne and its impact on the quality of life in school-aged adolescents in Malaysia. Journal of Primary Health Care. 2009;1(1):20–5.
9. Muthupalaniappen L, Tan HC, Puah JW, et al. Acne prevalence, severity and risk factors among medical students in Malaysia. Clin Ter 2014;165:187–92.
10. Hamilton, James B, Harumi Terada, and Gordon E. Mestler. "Greater Tendency to Acne in White American than in Japanese Populations 1." The Journal of Clinical Endocrinology & Metabolism 24.3 (1964): 267–72.

CHAPTER

4

Pathogenesis of Acne

Acne is a multifactorial disorder of the pilosebaceous unit. It presents clinically as mild comedonal acne to rarely fulminant systemic disease as acne fulminans. Sebaceous gland acts as peripheral endocrine unit and its role in acne pathogenesis is pivotal.

Acne primarily results from inflammation which is subclinical, resulting in formation of microcomedone at the level of isthmus of Sebaceous gland. Increased sebaceous gland secretions, alteration in quality of sebum lipids, regulation of cutaneous steroidogenesis, androgen activity, interaction with neuropeptides, follicular hyperkeratinization and the proliferation of *C. acnes* within the follicles are other complex factors which interplay in the etiology of acne.

ANATOMY OF SEBACEOUS GLAND

Sebaceous glands are unilobular or multilobular structures, usually associated with hair follicles. Sebum production occurs via **holocrine** secretion by the complete disintegration of the glandular cells (Fig. 4.1).

These are usually associated with a hair follicle except for **free sebaceous glands** found on vermilion border of lips, oral mucosa (**Fordyce** granules), eyelids (**meibomian** glands), areolae (**Montgomery** tubercles), labia minora and prepuce (**Tyson** glands). These produce sebum which is released into the infundibular portion of hair follicle. These glands are well-developed in scalp, face, upper back and chest, external auditory meatus and anogenital surfaces.

Pilosebaceous unit is made up of 4 parts: Keratinized follicular infundibulum, hair, sebaceous gland and sebaceous duct (Fig. 4.2).

Infundibulum has two parts:

1. Acroinfundibulum
2. Infrainfundibulum

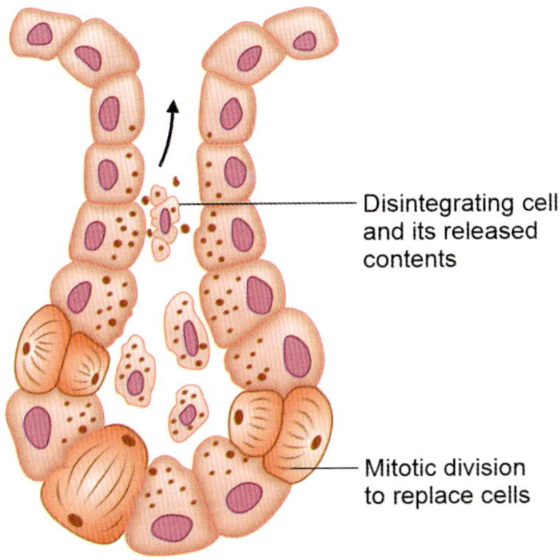

Fig. 4.1: Anatomy of sebaceous gland

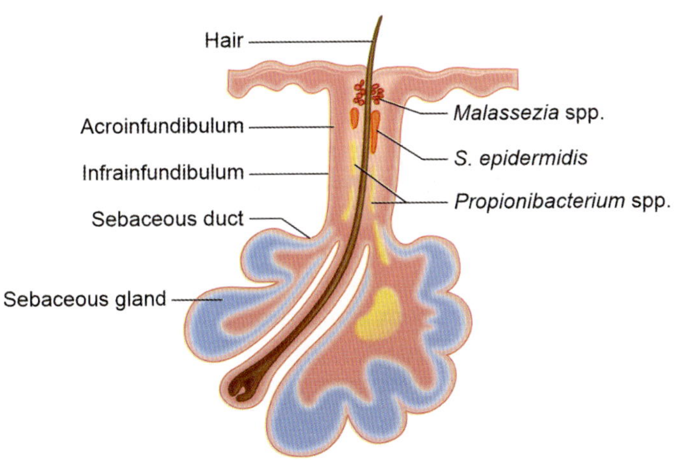

Fig. 4.2: Pilosebaceous unit

Malassezia spp., *Staph. epidermidis; Propionibacterium* spp. including *P. acnes, P. granulosum* and *P. parvum* are resident microflora within pilosebaceous unit. Recent key studies have highlighted a better understanding of the important role of *Cutibacterium acnes* (*C. acnes*) in the development of acne. Three major findings in the last decade include: (1) the ability of *C. acnes* to self-organize in a biofilm associated with a more virulent activity, (2) the loss of the *C. acnes* phylotype diversity, and (3) the central role of the T helper cell 17 pathway pathway in acne inflammation.[1]

Composition of Sebum

It is light yellow viscous fluid. Sebum contains triglycerides, free fatty acids, squalene, wax and sterol esters, and free sterols. During passage of sebum through the hair canal, bacterial enzymes hydrolyse some of the triglycerides so that the lipid mixture reaching the skin surface contains free fatty acids and small proportions of monoglycerides and diglycerides in addition to original components of sebum. Flow of the sebum is relatively continuous and sebocyte turnover time is approximately 14 days. The average rate of sebum production in adults is 1 mg/10 sq cm every 3 hr. Sebum production is relatively high at birth and it soon declines and remains low until puberty, at which time it rises again. The level of sebum production at the end of puberty remains constant through mid-adulthood.

Functions of Sebum

It reduces water loss from skin surface and keeps skin soft and smooth by maintaining stratum corneum hydration. It contains IgA, which protects the skin from infection by bacteria and fungi. Sebum flow to the surface of skin helps in vitamin E delivery to the upper skin layers, thereby protecting the skin and its surface lipids from oxidation. Androgens, retinoids, melanocortins, PPARs, fibroblast growth factor receptors, etc. are responsible for secretion and composition of sebum. Sebaceous gland requires androgenic stimulus in the form of **testosterone, DHT** and **DHEAS** to produce significant amount of sebum. It causes **increased sebocyte proliferation and increased lipid**

synthesis especially DHT. Individuals with a genetic deficiency of androgen receptors like in complete androgen insensitivity have no detectable sebum secretion and no acne.

Androgens, retinoids, melanocortins, PPARs, fibroblast growth factor receptors **affect sebaceous gland size and sebum production**.

CLASSICAL PATHOGENESIS OF ACNE

Acne Basically Results from

- Increased sebaceous gland activity with resultant seborrhea.
- Abnormal follicular differentiation with increased keratinization.
- Microbial hypercolonization of the follicular canal.
- Increased inflammation primarily through activation of adaptive immune system (Fig. 4.3).

Dietary Factors

The relationship between diet and acne remains still unproven. Studies have found that milk intake (especially skim milk) is positively associated with acne exacerbation. Dairy products contain 5-reduced steroid hormones and other steroid precursors of DHT6 that drive sebaceous gland function. Drinking milk causes a direct rise in IGF-1 through a disproportionate elevation in blood sugar and serum insulin levels.[2]

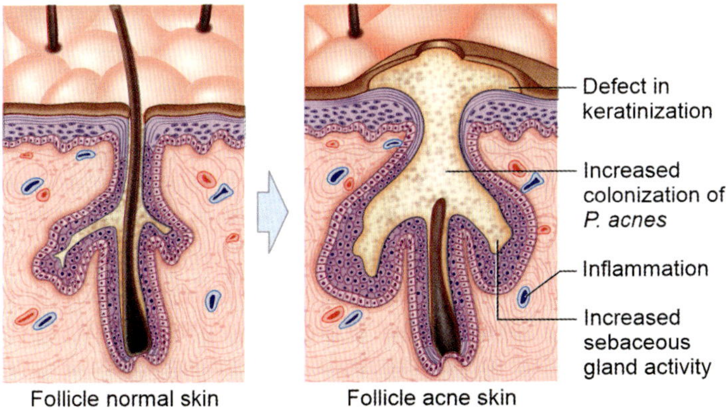

Fig. 4.3: Newer pathogenesis of acne

Vitamin A is needed for normal follicular function and is often deficient in teens. Supplementation of vitamin A in deficient persons helps in reducing plugging of pores. Dietary fatty acids influence inflammation, some are pro-inflammatory, some are anti-inflammatory, hence there is need for careful dietary selection for optimal disease control at least in a few cases.

Foods containing omega-3 essential fatty acids (EFAs) and EFA supplements may help to control inflammation and help in disease process indirectly. This signifies the importance of paleolithic diet in acne which includes consumption of vegetables, berries, seafish and green tea.

Genetic Factors

Usually acne runs in families. Association is observed in patients who have moderate to severe acne. Family history of acne is common but it is difficult to attribute only to genetic cause due to high prevalence of acne in the society.

Hyperkeratinization

It is one of the most crucial initial events in the development of acne. There are *in vitro* and *in vivo* studies which suggest IL-1 induce hyperkeratinization in follicular infundibulum (Fig. 4.4). In addition to this, there is a defect in the differentiation of infundibular keratinocytes, which is related to increased filaggrin (filament aggregating protein) expression. Hyperproliferation can be observed within infundibular keratinocytes, with the expression of the hyperproliferative markers keratin K6 and K16. IL-1 activates basal keratinocytes by autocrine production inducing K16 expression in supra-basal cells in the active state. Regarding the hormonal response, increased DHT may act on infundibular keratinocytes leading to abnormal hyperkeratinization. Follicular keratinization may be triggered by relative deficiency of linoleic acid and peroxides in sebum.

All these factors cause multiplication of keratinocytes and they are propelled towards the centre of the duct, which expands to accommodate the increasing bulk of the microcomedo until a point is reached beyond which the inelastic 'glassy membrane' that encloses the pilosebaceous duct can expand no further.

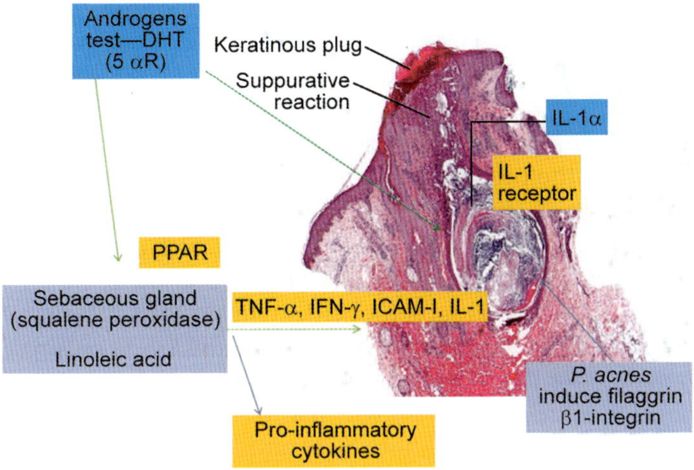

Fig. 4.4: Pathogenesis of acne

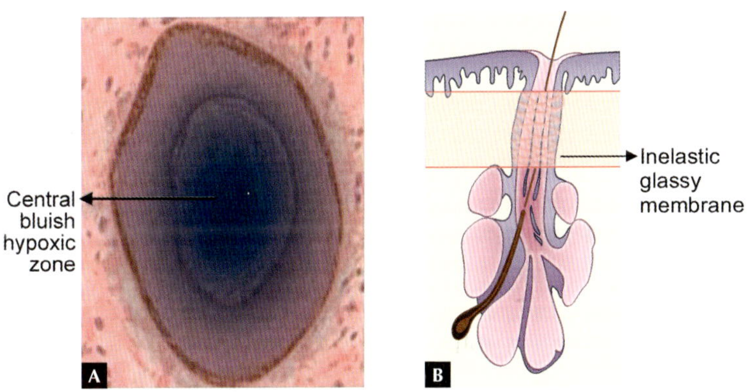

Fig. 4.5 A and B: Transverse section of pilosebaceous unit

Further production of keratinocytes into this closed system causes an increase in intraluminal pressure and this causes hypoxia centrally in the duct (Fig. 4.5 A and B). This produces an anoxic environment that favors development of intra-ductal *P. acnes* colonies. All these lead to rupture of the duct wall and inflammatory cascade begins.

Sebaceous Gland and Innate Immunity

Pilosebaceous unit is an immune-competent unit. Keratinocytes and sebocytes act as immune cells. They are capable of pathogen recognition, abnormal lipid presentation. Innate immunity includes molecules such as toll-like receptors TLR2 and TLR4, CD1d and CD14, antimicrobial peptides such as defensin-1, defensin-2 and cathelicidins. All these are expressed on sebocytes. They may recognize altered lipid content in sebum, followed by the production of inflammatory cytokines.

The monounsaturated fatty acids (MUFA), mainly palmitic acid (C16:1) and oleic acid (C18:1), both of which are bactericidal against Gram-positive organisms, are produced by the sebaceous gland, as is sapienic acid, an important antimicrobial lipid. Stearoyl coenzyme A desaturase (SCD) 1, an enzyme responsible for the biosynthesis of MUFA, is also expressed by the sebaceous gland. The TLR-2 ligand macrophage-activating lipopeptide- 2 stimulates both SCD and fatty acid desaturase-2 mRNA expression in SZ95 sebocytes.

Entry of Naïve Sebaceous Glands into the Acne Cycle: The Comedone Switch[3]

The initial key step for comedogenesis has been widely accepted to be an alteration of the epithelial wall of the infundibulum, particularly at the junction of the sebaceous gland duct (isthmus), with hyperproliferation of ductal keratinocytes and reduced separation of ductal corneocytes.

The causes of these alterations were believed to be:

- The comedogenic effects of certain sebaceous lipids.
- An androgen-controlled defect.
- Local cytokine modulation (interleukin-1 augments, epidermal growth factor prevents comedogenesis).
- Ductal bacteria, P. acnes, which results from hyperseborrhea and can generate both comedogenic lipids and the innate immunity cascade The Master Switch for Microcomedone Formation.

The master switch that transforms a normally functioning sebaceous gland into a microcomedone has been illustrated in Figure 4.6.

Topology of the Master Switch for Microcomedone Formation

It is accepted that the isthmus (the zone where the sebaceous gland duct joins the hair duct) is the zone where the microcomedone

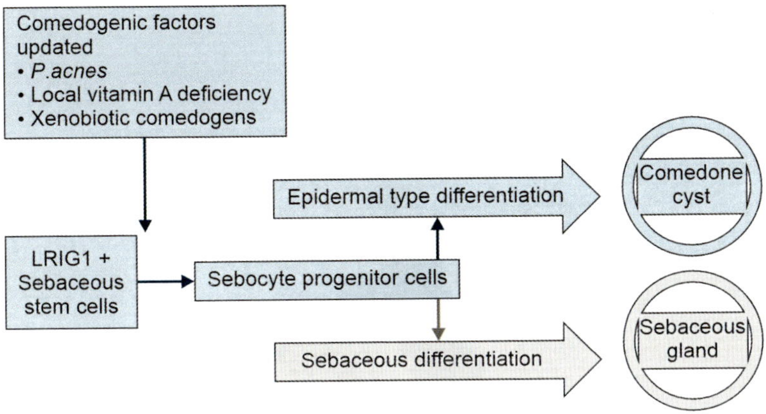

Fig. 4.6: The comedone switch in the differentiation of sebaceous gland stem cells

develops. Leucine-rich repeats and immunoglobulin-like domains protein-1 (LRIG1) cells contributes to the epithelium of the isthmus and populates sebaceous glands (Fig. 4.7). LRIG cells may therefore differentiate toward either an epithelial type or a sebaceous type and should therefore be primary targets for comedogenic factors (Fig. 4.6).

In summary, this scenario offers a simple master switch model for comedone formation that articulates the different etiological agents as well as the potential mode of action of therapeutic and preventive interventions.

Preventing the Comedone Switch?

1. Ductal *P. acnes* control may be obtained primarily by reducing sebum production, which feeds the bacterial growth. This may account for the effect of oral isotretinoin and topical retinoids. Topical agent with a significant sebum suppressive effect, and clean safety profile for long-term use, would appear as a 'disease-modifying' breakthrough compound. Topical retinoid therapy appears to act towards restoring adequate retinoid signaling in the infundibulum/isthmus epithelium, and this should prevent the abnormal differentiation resulting in the comedone switch and stem cell commitment.
2. Ductal *P. acnes* control also obtained by oral and topical antibiotics.

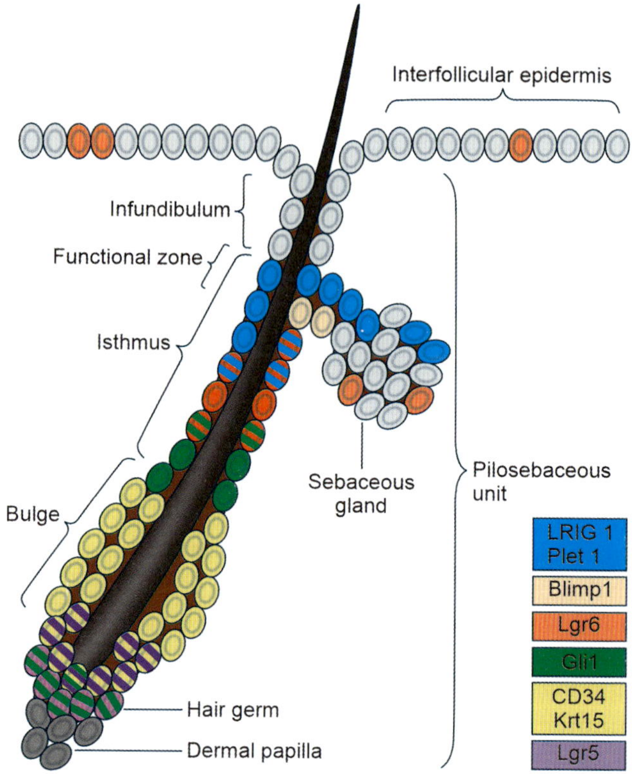

Fig. 4.7: Different stem cell populations are shown in the mouse resting (telogen) adult hair follicle. Each stem cell compartment is defined by distinct protein expression and gene promoter activity; cells with multiple colors express multiple markers

Topical retinoid use should therefore be revisited as targeting acne-prone normal-looking skin in a preventive dimension, rather than just only as comedolytic.

Thus, the key target for acne care is naïve follicles that is not involved yet to prevent comedone switch.

ROLE OF TOLL-LIKE RECEPTORS

Toll-like receptors (TLRs) are a group of pattern recognition receptors. They recognize pathogen-associated molecular patterns (PAMPs). They are trans-membrane proteins responsible for innate immune response against bacteria. TLR stimulation promotes the production of proinflammatory cytokines, prostaglandins, leukotrienes (LT) and chemokines.

P. acnes activate TLR-2, resulting in increased levels of IL-8, IL-12, tumor necrosis factor-α, and IL-1β. All-trans retinoic acid specifically downregulate the cell surface expression of TLR-2 and CD14.

FGFR1 and FGFR2 are expressed in epidermis and skin appendages. FGFR3 and FGFR4 are localized in dermal vessels and absent in epidermis and skin appendages.

Insulin-like growth factor-1 can induce sterol response binding protein-1 (SREBP-1), which stimulates sebaceous gland lipogenesis.

Substance P (SP) is found to be expressed in dermal nerves around the sebaceous glands of acne patients. It promotes proliferation and the differentiation of sebaceous glands and increases immune reactivity and RNA expression of proinflammatory cytokines.

Facial sebum from acne patients contain MMP-1, MMP-13, TIMP-1 and TIMP-2, which originate in keratinocytes and sebocytes. *P. acnes* induces MMP-9, MMP-1, and TIMP-1 transcription in human monocytes. MMP-1, -2, -3, and -9 are significantly upregulated in acne lesions. The upregulated MMPs contribute to the acne pathogenesis by inducing inflammation and tissue destruction. Having role in the skin's immune defence system by direct microbial toxicity and also by modulating components of innate and adaptive immune systems.

Anti-microbial peptides are produced by keratinocytes, monocytes, mast cells, sebocytes, neutrophils and natural killer cells. **They are cathelicidins, [beta]-defensins and granulysin**.

Peroxisome proliferator activated receptors are orphan nuclear receptors similar to retinoid receptors. Peroxisome proliferator-activated receptors (PPARs) are ligand-activated transcription factors involved in the genetic regulation of the lipid metabolism and energy homeostasis. There is increased sebum production and inflammation due to their effect on lipid deposition in the sebocytes and inhibition of proinflammatory gene expression and downregulation of inflammatory cytokines. In patients receiving fibrates (PPAR-alpha ligand) for hyperlipidemia and thiazolidinediones (PPAR-gamma ligand) for diabetes, sebum secretion rate is increased. Activation of PPAR-α appears to increase differentiation-induced apoptosis, contribute to follicular comedogenesis.

Activation of PPAR-gamma by UV-B irradiation and potent lipid soluble oxidant induces COX-2 expression in SZ95 sebocytes and causes sebocyte proliferation and/or lipogenesis. Human sebocytes express all necessary enzymes for a functional leukotriene pathway. The enzymes 5-LOX and LTA4 hydrolase are expressed in SZ95 sebocytes at protein and mRNA level which are essential for formation of LTB4. LTB4 is also a natural ligand for peroxisome proliferator-activated receptor PPAR. Treatment of S95 sebocytes with AA stimulates 5-LOX expression and induces LTB4 synthesis in addition, it also induces IL6 and IL8 which aggravates acne. Thus involvement of 5-LOX in pathogenesis of acne has led to role of newer medication like LOX inhibitor zileuton (inhibit leukotrienes B4) in acne management.

Recent evidence of the anti-apoptotic effect of the PPAR-agonist, rosiglitazone on SZ-95 sebocytes *in vitro* (thereby inhibiting the final step in holocrine secretion of sebum), thereby making PPAR ligands as future options in acne management.

Clinical lesion of acne is determined by type of immunological response. Neutrophils predominate in early stage of acne which leads to formation of suppurative pustules. Lymphocytes predominate in later stages which leads to formation of inflamed papules, nodules, and cysts. Scarring in acne patients is determined by severity of inflammation.

Inflammation basically precedes hyperproliferation as per newer hypothesis. There is an increase in IL-1 activity and number of CD4+ before hyperproliferation around uninvolved follicles which ultimately trigger activation of keratinocytes. Most common up regulated genes involved in acne lesions are matrix metalloproteinase, human beta defensin 4, IL-8, granulysin. Nuclear factor kappa which is a transcription factor upregulating many proinflammatory genes.

Studies suggest that TNF-α induces lipogenesis in SZ95 sebocytes through JNK pathways. IL-1β is abundant in inflammatory acne lesions. Inflammation is further characterised by action of active lipid mediators like leukotrienes, prostaglandins and 15-hydroxyeicosatetraenoic acid. Now new research suggests pivotal role of Th17.

COX2 expression is selectively upregulated in acne involving sebaceous glands. Further activation of platelet activating factors which consist of a group of phosphocholines with various biological effects, like modulation of keratinocyte function and skin inflammation. Transgenic keratin 5 promoter driven over-expression of COX2, increases PGE2 level resulting into sebaceous gland hyperplasia as well as increased sebum production.

NEUROPHYSIOLOGY[4]

Human skin particularly sebaceous gland expresses functional receptors for neuropeptides such as corticotropin releasing hormone the most proximal element of hypothalamic pituitary adrenal axis, melanocortins, β-endorphins, vasoactive intestinal polypeptide, neuropeptide Y and calcitonin gene-related peptide.[5]

These receptors modulate the production of inflammatory cytokines, proliferation, differentiation, lipogenesis and androgen metabolism in human sebocytes.

IMPORTANCE OF CAUSATIVE ORGANISM IN PATHOGENESIS: *Propionibacterium acnes*

Propionibacterium acnes contribute significantly to the pathogenesis of acne. These are found within sebaceous follicle. These are anaerobic/microaerophilic, Gram-positive, non-motile rods. These naturally produce porphyrins (primarily coproporphyrin III) that fluorescence under Wood's lamp illumination. Bacteria have single circular chromosome. Genes code for host tissue degradation enzymes with five Christie-Atkins-Munch-Petersen (CAMP) factors, acting as 2 nm membrane pore-forming toxin and proteins for biofilm synthesis.

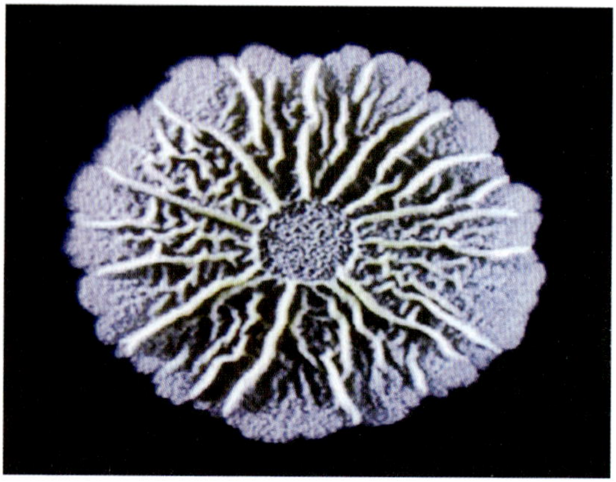

Fig. 4.8: Biofilm

Biofilm is glycocalyx polymer, which serves as a biological glue between keratinocytes and also limiting effective antimicrobial concentrations within the biofilm microenvironment and promoting antibiotic resistance (Fig. 4.8).

Interactions between the skin's innate immune system and *P. acnes* play an important role in acne pathogenesis. *P. acnes* have been shown to stimulate the release of proinflammatory mediators (e.g. IL-1α, IL-8, IL-12, tumor necrosis factor-α [TNF-α], matrix metalloproteinases) through the toll-like receptor 2 and 4 pathway (Figs 4.9 and 4.10).

IL-8 results in neutrophil recruitment, the release of lysosomal enzymes and subsequent disruption of the follicular epithelium. *P. acnes* strains modulate expression of immune markers at both gene and protein formation level.

The adaptive immune response has a central role in the inflammation observed in acne, resulting from the recruitment of activated T helper 1 (Th1) cells and Th17 cells.

Th17 cells are characterized by the production of IL-17A and IL-17F belonging to the IL-17 family of cytokines. IL-17A and IL-17 F target mostly non-lymphoid cells including fibroblasts, keratinocytes, endothelial cells, and macrophages, and induce the production of cytokines such as TNF-α, IL-6, GM-CSF, and matrix metalloproteinases. In addition to IL-17A and F, Th17 cells produce IL-6, IL-21, and IL-22 and

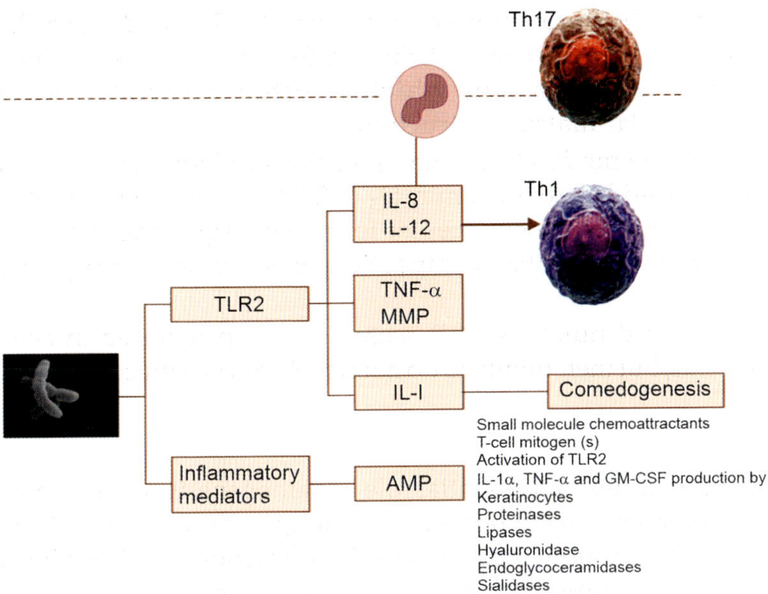

Fig. 4.9: Role of inflammatory mediators

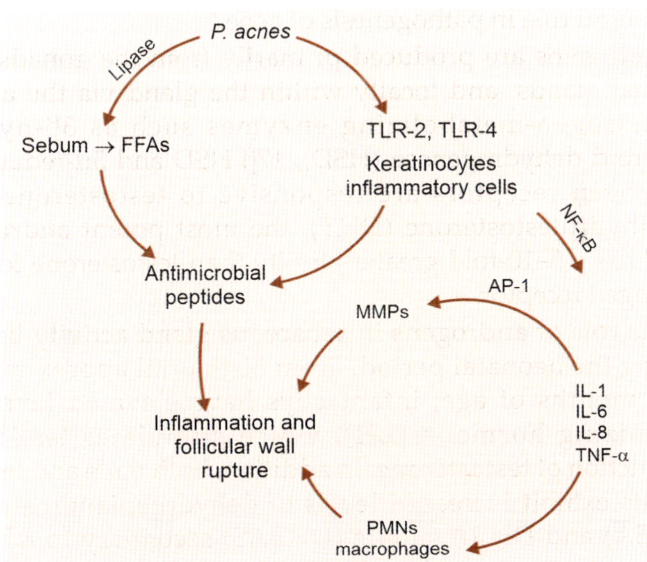

Fig. 4.10: Pathogenesis of acne by *P. acnes*

exhibit effector functions distinct from the Th1 and Th2 cells. An important outcome of these effects is localized chronic tissue inflammation, which is often associated with extracellular matrix destruction.

Immune modulators such as all-trans retinoic acid (ATRA) and 1, 25-dihydroxyvitamin D_3 ($1,25D_3$) share the retinoid X receptor as a common receptor for retinoid signaling and have been tried as potential therapeutic agents in inflammatory acne lesions.

Increased numbers of *P. acnes* have been reported in acne patients, but their numbers do not correlate with clinical severity.

HORMONES

Androgens play an essential role in pathogenesis of acne, most of the patients have normal circulating androgen level. Acne severity does not correlate with it. Sebaceous gland has been shown to express all necessary enzymes for biosynthesis of testosterone *de novo* from cholesterol and substances ingested like dairy products.[6] Hormonal effects on sebum secretion have the central role in pathogenesis of acne.[7]

Androgens are produced primarily from the gonads and adrenal glands, and locally within the gland via the action of androgen-metabolizing enzymes such as 3β-hydroxysteroid dehydrogenase (HSD), 17β-HSD and 5α-reductase. Androgen receptors are responsive to testosterone and 5α-dihydrotestosterone (DHT), the most potent androgen. DHT has a 5–10-fold greater affinity than testosterone for the androgen receptor.

The role of androgens in sebaceous gland activity begins during the neonatal period. From birth until approximately 6–12 months of age, infant boys have elevated levels of luteinizing hormone (LH), which stimulates testicular production of testosterone. In addition, both male and female infants exhibit increased levels of dehydroepiandrosterone (DHEA) and DHEA sulfate (DHEAS) secondary to a large, androgen producing "fetal zone" in the adrenal gland that involutes over 1 year of life. Both testicular and adrenal androgen production decrease substantially by 1 year of age and remain at a stable nadir until adrenarche. With the onset of adrenarche (typically at 7–8 years of age, usually heralding menarche by several years), circulating levels of DHEA-S begin to rise due to adrenal production. This hormone can serve as a precursor for the synthesis of more potent androgens within the sebaceous gland. The rise in serum levels of DHEA-S in pre-pubescent children is associated with an increase in sebum production and the initial development of comedonal acne.[8]

The main influence of androgens is on the proliferation and differentiation of keratinocytes. Androgen receptors are present in the basal layer of the sebaceous gland and the outer root sheath of the hair follicle. DHT has the capability of binding to and activating its intranuclear receptor; however, this receptor is regulated by the transcription factor, Forkhead box protein O1 (FoxO1). The regulatory capacity of FoxO1 is inhibited by the protein kinase Akt, a downstream target associated with insulin- and insulin-like growth factor-1 (IGF-1)-receptor activation. Transient rises of insulin and IGF-1 occurring during the normal course of puberty inhibit FoxO1 regulation and allow the activated androgen receptor to trigger a chain of metabolic events, which lead to an excess production of keratinocytes and sebum. This process is augmented by the additional regulatory duty of Akt on TSC1/2, an inhibitor of mTOR, where its inactivation allows mammalian perform its downstream signaling duties, which will inevitably lead to the increase of lipid and protein synthesis within the PSU (Fig. 4.11).

DHT has sebocytes proliferation effect which is mediated by SZ95 sebocyte differentiation and lipogenesis which is due to upregulation of sterol response element binding protein (SREBP). Comedogenesis is due to DHT action which leads to hyperkeratinisation of infrainfundibular canal.

While the occurrence of acne vulgaris in males and females is initiated by the onset of puberty, it is most likely prolonged into late adolescence by transient increases in insulin and IGF-1 levels.[9]

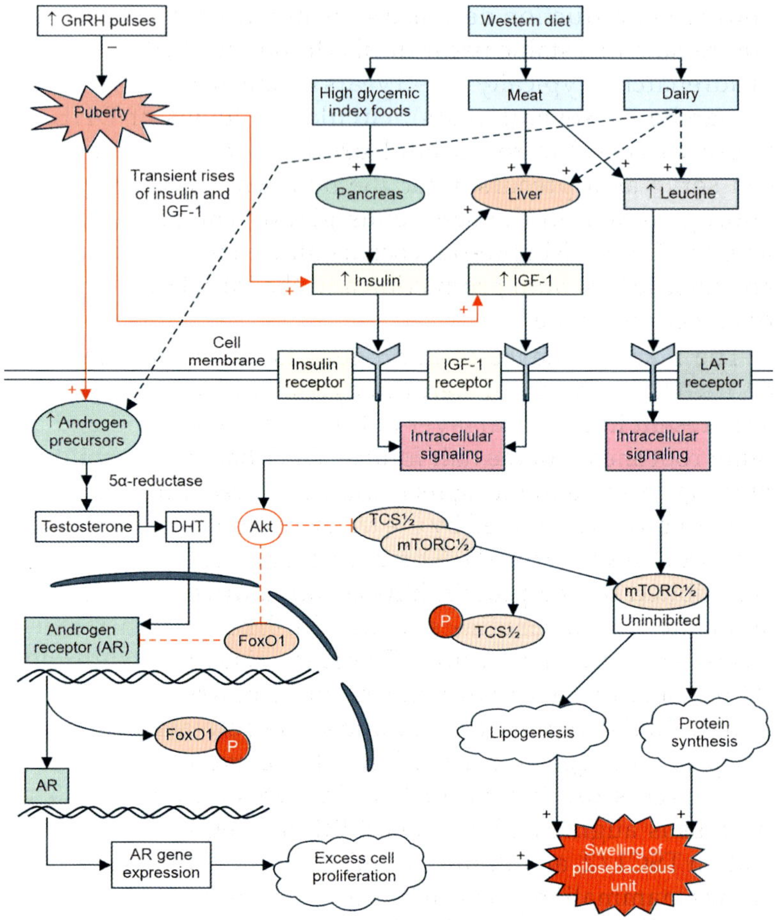

Fig. 4.11: Cellular mechanisms hypothesized to govern the pathogenesis of acne vulgaris.

GnRH: Gonadotropin-releasing hormone; *IGF:* Insulin growth factor; *DHT:* Dihydrotestosterone; *FoxO1:* Forkhead box protein O1; *mTORC:* mammalian target of rapamycin

REFERENCES

1. Mias C, Mengeaud V, Bessou-Touya S, Duplan H. Recent advances in understanding inflammatory acne: Deciphering the relationship between Cutibacterium acnes and Th17 inflammatory pathway. Journal of the European Academy of Dermatology and Venereology. 2023 Mar;37:3–11.

2. Darling JA, Laing AH, Harkness RA. A survey of the steroids in cows'milk. Journal of Endocrinology. 1974 Aug;62(2):291–7.
3. Saurat JH. Strategic targets in acne: The comedone switch in question. Dermatology. 2015 Jul;231(2):105–11.
4. Kurokawa I, Danby FW, Ju Qiang, et al. New developments in our understanding of acne pathogenesis and treatment. Exp Dermatol 2009; 18:821–32. Cross Ref link Pubmed link.
5. Freedberg IM, Tomic Canic M, Komine M, Blumenberg M. Keratins and the keratinocyte activation cycle. J Invest Dermatol 2001;116: 633–40. Cross Ref link Pubmed link.
6. Albuquerque RG, Rocha MA, Bagatin E, et al. Could adult female acne be associated with modern life? Arch Dermatol Res. 2014;306:683–8. Cross Ref link Pubmed link.
7. Chen W, Tsai S J, Liao C Y, et al. Higher levels of steroidogenic acute regulatory protein and type I 3 beta-hydroxysteroid dehydrogenase in the scalp of men with androgenetic alopecia. J Invest Dermatol 2006: 126: 2332–5.
8. Lucky AW, Biro FM, Husten GA, et al. Acne vulgaris in premenstrual girls. An early stage of puberty associated with rising level of DHEA Arch Dermatol. 1994;130:308–14.
9. Lynn DD, Umari T, Dunnick CA, Dellavalle RP. The epidemiology of acne vulgaris in late adolescence. Adolescent Health, Medicine and Therapeutics. 2016:13–25.

CHAPTER 5

Clinical Manifestations of Acne

Acne usually begins with the onset of puberty. Acne is typically found on sites with well-developed sebaceous glands, mostly affecting the face, but it may involve the neck, chest and back, upper arms and may even occur extensively over the body. The lesions are centered on the pilosebaceous unit, i.e. the hair follicle and its associated oil gland which is stimulated by androgens. The lesions can be non-inflammatory or inflammatory. The initial lesions are usually non-inflammatory and centro-facial. With maturation inflammatory lesions may appear, involving face and even the trunk.

Severity of acne is variable but can be clearly correlated with the stage of puberty.

ACNE GRADING

1. Three Category System

Acne may be classified as mild, moderate or severe. Comedones and inflammatory lesions are usually considered separately.

Mild Acne

- <20 comedones
- <15 inflammatory lesions
- Or, total lesion count is <30

Moderate Acne

- 20–100 comedones
- 15–50 inflammatory lesions
- Or, total lesion count is 30–125

Severe Acne

- >5 pseudocysts
- Total comedo count >100
- Total inflammatory count >50
- Or total lesion count >125

Clinical Grading of Acne[1]

- **Grade 1:** Comedones, occasional papules
- **Grade 2:** Papules, comedones, a few pustules
- **Grade 3:** Mainly pustules, nodules and abscesses
- **Grade 4:** Mainly cysts or abscesses, scarring

2. Leeds Revised Acne Grading System

Used for research purposes, provides a photographic standard for acne grading of the face, back and chest.[2]

It includes:

- 15 facial grades (three solely for comedonal acne)
- 8 each for the chest and back.

However, this system does not adequately differentiate those with milder acne.[3]

3. Global Acne Grading System (GAGS)[1]

It is quantitative scoring system; involving summation of six regional subscores.[4]

Location	*Factor*
Forehead	2
Right cheek	2
Left cheek	2
Nose	1
Chin	1
Chest and upper back	3

Where
0 = no lesions
1 = comedones
2 = papules

3 = pustules
4 = nodules

4. Investigators' Global Assessment (IgGA) Scale

Given by Allen and Smith Jr; based on descriptive text of five categories but allowed for nine acne grades.

5. Acne Grading Method by Cook, et al.

Acne grading method by Cook, et al.,[1] using photographic standards.

Grade	*Description*
0	Up to 3 small scattered comedones and/or small papules are allowed.
2	Very few pustules or 3 dozens papules and/or comedones; lesions are hardly visible from 2.5 m away.
4	There are red lesions and inflammation to a significant degree; worthy of treatment.
6	Loaded with comedones, numerous pustules; lesions are easily recognized at 2.5 m.
8	Conglobata, sinus or cystic type acne; covering most of the face.

6. Five-category Global System

Given by US-FDA; includes detailed descriptive text.

- Clear, indicating no inflammatory or non-inflammatory lesions.
- Almost clear, rare non-inflammatory lesions with no more than one papule/pustule.
- Mild, some non-inflammatory lesions, no more than a few papules/pustules but no nodules.
- Moderate, up to many non-inflammatory lesions, may have some inflammatory lesions, but no more than one small nodule.
- Severe, up to many non-inflammatory and inflammatory lesions, but no more than a few nodules.

7. Comprehensive-acne Severity System[3]

Comprehensive-acne severity system (CASS) was developed by application of a pre-existing six-category facial investigator

Table 5.1: Comprehensive acne severity system

Grade	*Description*	*Face*	*Back*	*Chest*
Clear	No lesions to barely noticeable ones. Very few scattered comedones and papules			
Almost clear	Hardly visible from 2.5 m away. A few scattered comedones, a few small papules and very pustules			
Mild	Easily recognizable, less than half the affected area involved. Many comedones, papules and pustules			
Moderate	More than half the affected area involved. Numerous comedones, papules and pustules			
Severe	Entire area affected. Covered with comedones, papules and pustules and a few nodules and cysts			
Very severe	Highly inflammatory acne covering the affected area, with nodules and cysts present			

global assessment scale ranging from clear through to very severe grading. It is a very useful tool to compare treatment outcomes (Table 5.1).

8. Acne-specific Quality-of-life (QOL) Scales[5]

The use of QOL measures captures the impact of acne and treatment on the patient's life and helps to identify those vulnerable to psychological complications. Disease-specific questionnaires that relate specifically to acne include the Cardiff Acne Disability Index (CADI), the Assessment of the Psychosocial Effects of Acne (APSEA), the Acne Quality of Life Scale (Acne-QOL) and the Acne Quality-of-life four-item index (Acne-Q4).

COMEDONES

Comedones are early non-inflammatory lesions of acne. The precursor lesion is a microcomedo which cannot be perceived clinically occur because of blockage of the hair follicle.

Microcomedo evolves into open or closed comedone and further into papule or nodule.

Open Comedones (Blackheads)

These are dome-shaped papules having a dilated follicular opening which is filled with shed keratin. These have propensity to develop in midfacial region but can be seen in other acne prone areas as well. When evident early, these indicate poor prognosis. These are black may be because of oxidation of melanin or due to some lipids in sebum. Open comedones rarely become inflamed unlike closed comedones (whiteheads) which frequently become inflamed (Fig. 5.1).

Closed Comedones (Whiteheads)

Closed comedones (1 mm) are skin-colored papules with no apparent follicular opening. These are subtle and better appreciated upon palpation, stretching or side-lighting of the skin (Fig. 5.1).

Subtypes of comedones have been described as:

- **'Sandpaper' comedones:** Multiple very small whiteheads, over forehead produce a roughened, gritty feel to the skin.

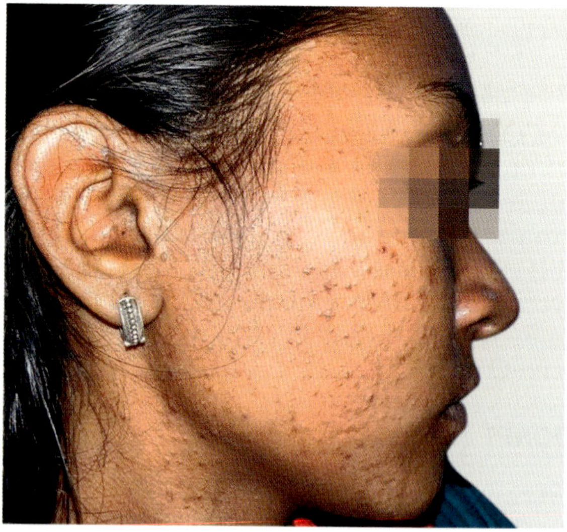

Fig. 5.1: Open and closed comedones (grade 1)

- **'Macrocomedones':** Large whiteheads greater than 1 mm in diameter.
- **'Submarine' comedones (>0.5 cm, large and deep):** Reside more deeply in the skin; and are frequently associated with recurrent inflammatory nodular lesions.
- **'Secondary' comedones:**[6] On exposure to topical steroids, pomade (pomade acne), thick oils and chemicals.
- Solar comedones or senile comedones are thought to be due to sun damage; found over the cheeks and chin of older people (Also known as "Favre-Racouchot" syndrome or solar elastosis).
- **Missed comedones:**[7] Comedones which are missed when not visualized with skin stretching or under good lighting.
- **Nevoid comedones:**[8] It is a rare condition considered to be a type of epidermal nevus. It presents as grouped, dilated follicular openings with dark keratin plugs (Fig. 5.2).
- **Double-ended comedones/Pseudocomedones (DEPs):**[9] DEPs are keratin-filled interconnected multipores and are considered a typical sign of HS.

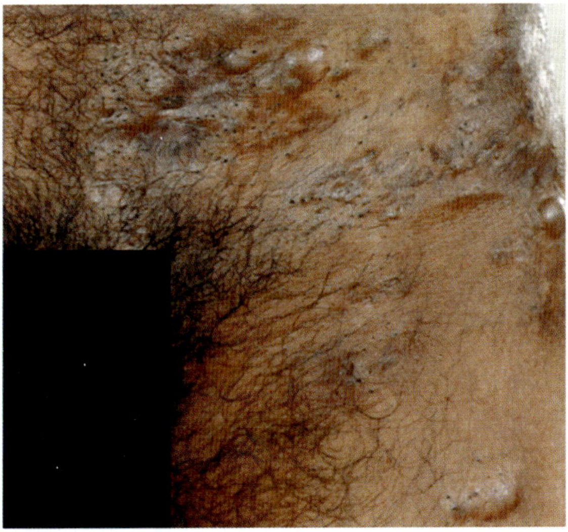

Fig. 5.2: Nevoid comedones/Nevus comedonicus

PAPULES

Papules (1 to 5 mm) are caused by the rupture of the follicle wall resulting in an inflammatory response (Fig. 5.3).

PUSTULE

A pustule (1 to 5 mm) is a pus-filled lesion and resolves in around five days, or longer (Fig. 5.4).

NODULOCYSTIC ACNE

Nodules are painful lesions that are greater than 5 mm in size and they can cause scarring. A cyst is deeper closed cavity having either pus or keratin. In severe nodulocystic acne, these lesions may coalesce to form large inflamed plaques that can include sinus tracts. These lesions are very tender, chronic and more resistant to treatment (Fig. 5.5).

Secondary Lesions

Erythema, post-inflammatory hyperpigmentation and scars often persist after resolution of inflammatory acne lesions.

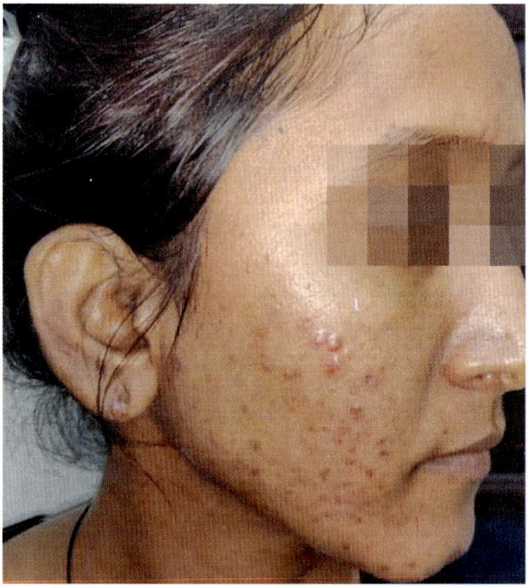

Fig. 5.3: Inflammatory papules over right cheek of an adolescent girl (grade 2)

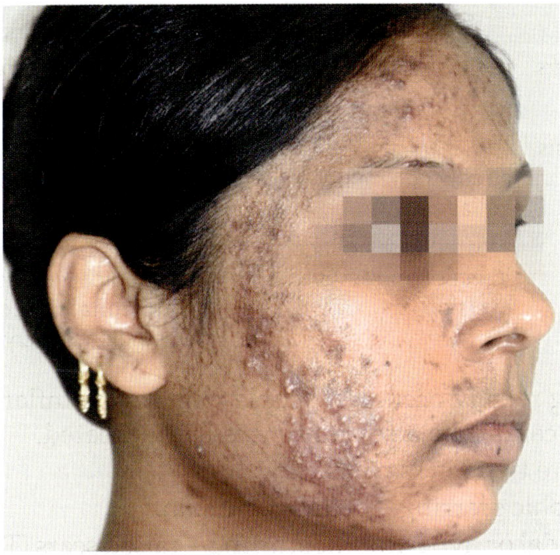

Fig. 5.4: Papules and pustules over right cheek (grade 3)

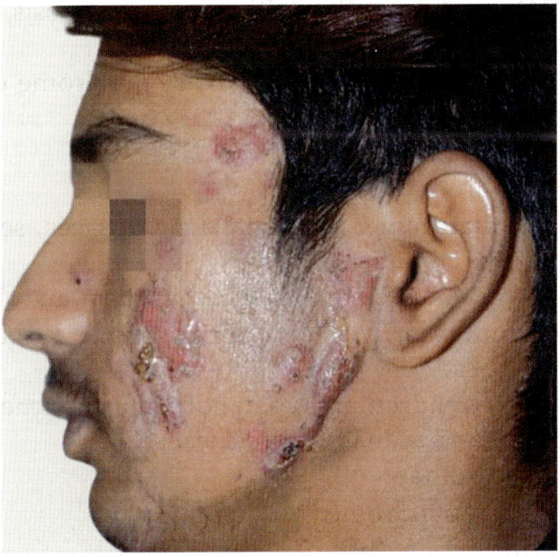

Fig. 5.5: Nodulocystic lesions over left cheek (grade 4)

Post-inflammatory hyperpigmentation is very common in racially pigmented patients.

Table 5.2: Difference between atrophic and keloidal scars		
Type of scars	*Atrophic scars*	*Keloidal or hypertrophic scars*
Incidence	More common	Less common
Pathogenesis	These are caused by a reduced amount of collagen	These are caused by an increase in the amount of collagen
Treatment	Treated with collagen injection or removed by excision	These scars can be treated with potent topical corticosteroids, intralesional injections of triamcinolone, or cryotherapy.

Scarring mostly occurs in people with severe inflammatory acne or in cases where severe acne is left untreated.

There are two kinds of scarring:[2]

- Atrophic scarring—beneath the skin.
- Keloidal or hypertrophic scarring—raised scars (Table 5.2).

Acne Associated Diseases Include

- **SAPHO syndrome:** Synovitis, acne, pustulosis, hyperostosis, and osteitis.[4]
- **PCOS syndrome:** Polycystic ovary syndrome or Stein-Leventhal syndrome.
- PAPASH syndrome
- PASH syndrome
- **MARSH syndrome:** Melasma, acne, rosacea, seborrheic eczema and Hirsutism.[10]
- **SAHA syndrome:** Seborrhea, acne, hirsutism, and alopecia.[11]
- **PAPA syndrome:** Pyogenic arthritis, pyoderma gangrenosum, and acne.
- **HAIR-AN syndrome:** Hyperandrogenism, acne, insulin resistance, and acanathosis nigricans.
- Apert syndrome.[12]
- Klinefelter's syndrome.[13]
- Pyoderma gangrenosum.[6]

REFERENCES

1. Adityan B, Kumari R, Thappa DM. Scoring systems in acne vulgaris. Indian J Dermatol Venereol Leprol 2009;75:323–6.

2. McWilliam J. Acne vulgaris: clinical features, assessment and treatment. Nursing Standard. 2009:23, 34, 49–56.
3. Tan JK, Tang J, Fung K, Gupta AK, Thomas DR, Sapra S, Lynde C, Poulin Y, Gulliver W, Sebaldt RJ. Development and validation of a comprehensive acne severity scale. Journal of Cutaneous Medicine and Surgery. 2007 Nov;11(6):211–6.
4. Pons, Jean-Claude, Larissa Nekhlyudov, and Jean-François Delfraissy. "The course of the SAPHO syndrome during pregnancy." European Journal of Obstetrics and Gynecology and Reproductive Biology 70.2 (1996): 215–6.
5. The Cardiff Acne Disability Index. Br J Dermatol, 2021;185:e161-e161. https://doi.org/10.1111/bjd.20671.
6. Shenefelt PD. Pyoderma gangrenosum associated with cystic acne and hidradenitis suppurativa controlled by adding minocycline and sulfasalazine to the treatment regimen. Cutis 57.5 (1996): 315–9.
7. Cunliffe WJ, Holland DB, Clark SM, Stables GI. Comedogenesis: some new aetiological, clinical and therapeutic strategies. British Journal of Dermatology. 2000 Jun;142(6):1084–91.
8. Tchernev G, Ananiev J, Semkova K, Dourmishev LA, Schönlebe J, Wollina U. Nevus comedonicus: an updated review. Dermatology and therapy. 2013 Jun;3:33–40.
9. Lee EY, Alhusayen R, Lansang P, Shear N, Yeung J. What is hidradenitis suppurativa? Can Fam Physician. 2017;63(2):114-120. PMID: 28209676; PMCID: PMC5395382.
10. Griffiths D. The red face—an overview and delineation of the MARSH syndrome. Clinical and experimental dermatology. 1999 Jan;24(1):42–7.
11. Orfanos Constantin E, Yael D. Adler, Christos CZ. The SAHA syndrome. Hormone Research in Paediatrics 54.5-6 (2000): 251–8.
12. Henderson CA et al. Apert's syndrome and androgen receptor staining of the basal cells of sebaceous glands. British Journal of Dermatology 132.1 (1995): 139–43.
13. Wollenberg A et al. Acne conglobata and Klinefelter's syndrome. British Journal of Dermatology 136.3 (1997): 421–3.

CHAPTER

6

Systemic Associations of Acne

INTRODUCTION

Acne is a chronic disease and a reflection of disturbances of hormonal and, at times, immunological milieu. Appropriate hormonal evaluation of all cases of atypical acne is ideally required.

An understanding of dermato-endocrinology, in terms of pathogenetic mechanisms of hormonal acne, methodology of hormonal assays and their fallacies will allow early diagnosis of the root cause.

EPIDEMIOLOGY

Indian women have a higher degree of hirsutism, infertility, and acne as compared to women of Caucasian ethnicity. Acne and oily skin (40.6 *vs.* 22.6%) is significantly higher in obese than lean polycystic ovary syndrome (PCOS) women.[1]

PATHOGENESIS

Stratum granulosum is the site for conversion of inactive precursors to potent androgen, so there is increased local androgen bioactivity (Fig. 6.1). 80% of testosterone is bound to sex hormone-binding globulin (SHBG), 19% is bound to albumin, and 1% circulates freely in blood stream. Testosterone is acted upon by 5-alpha reductase into dihydrotestosterone (DHT), which is 5–10 times more potent than testosterone. Excess androgen, insulin and IGF-1 give a positive feedback to the enzyme and hence the level of DHT increases. Androgenicity depends mainly on unbound

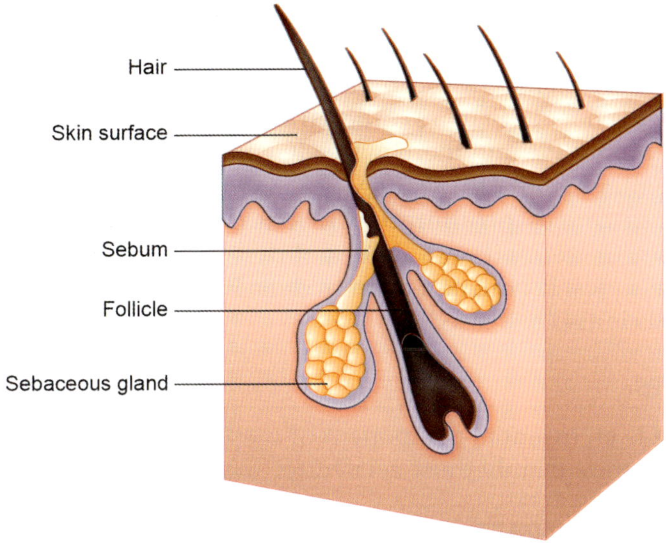

Fig. 6.1: Peripheral metabolism of androgens: Skin and pilosebaceous unit

fraction as it interacts with receptors. If SHBG levels are increased, the free androgen reduces and if SHBG levels are reduced, the free androgen increases causing androgen related effects on the body. Although the blood levels are not high, the local androgen activity is increased. Skin is an important peripheral site for androgen production in women (Table 6.1).[2, 3]

Androgens and insulin/IGF-1 determine androgen receptor activity. Only testosterone and DHT are able to activate androgen receptors which promote sebum production and inflammation.

Insulin and androgen metabolism are interlinked. Hyperinsulinemia causes increase in serum levels of IGF-1. IGF may stimulate comedogenic factors—androgen. Incidence of acne

Table 6.1: Source of circulating androgens in females[4]

Site	*Testosterone (%)*	*DHEA (%)*	*Androstenedione (%)*	*DHEAS (%)*
Ovaries	20	20	50	—
Adrenals	25	80	50	100

corresponds more closely to insulin and IGF-1 levels than plasma androgens.

Insulin increases the bioavailability of sex steroids (by reducing hepatic SHBG synthesis) and inhibits synthesis of IGF binding protein and thereby free IGF increases.

Insulin also increases hepatic production of IGF-1, which in turn causes proliferation of basal keratinocytes in the pilosebaceous unit and abnormal desquamation of follicular corneocytes. Production of androgens by gonadal and adrenal glands is also increased.

TYPES

Acne is an essential component of many systemic diseases or syndromes, mainly those related to:[5]

Androgen or Insulin Excess or "Hormonal Acne"

Androgen excess may be due to the following causes:

a. Polycystic ovarian syndrome (PCOS)
b. Congenital adrenal hyperplasia (CAH)
c. Seborrhea, acne, hirsutism androgenetic alopecia (SAHA) syndrome
d. Hyperandrogenism, acne, insulin resistance, acanthosis nigricans (HAIR-AN) syndrome.

Autoinflammatory Conditions

These lead to IL-1 abnormalities. Examples are:

a. Synovitis-acne-pustulosis-hyperostosis-osteitis (SAPHO) syndrome
b. Pyogenic arthritis, pyoderma gangrenosum, acne (PAPA) syndrome, PAPASH syndrome, and
c. Apert syndrome.

POLYCYSTIC OVARIAN SYNDROME

Polycystic ovarian syndrome (PCOS) is a common, complex, heterogeneous endocrine disorder affecting 5 to 20% of women. It is characterized by clinical and/or biochemical evidence of hyperandrogenism with oligo- and/or anovulation and polycystic ovaries and a metabolic derangement including glucose intolerance and hyperinsulinemia.[6]

Obesity is present in 30–75% of women with PCOS, however, lean PCOS is also becoming common. Sedentary lifestyle is associated with increased metabolic dysfunction. Strong genetic background is seen in many cases.

Clinical Features

PCOS varies at various life stages. In adolescent period, it manifests with menstrual irregularity and cosmetic concerns like acne, hirsutism, hair loss. During reproductive period, it may cause infertility and during pregnancy complications like pregnancy-induced hypertersion (PIH), gestational diabetes (GDM), and early pregnancy loss may occur.

At menopause, it causes metabolic syndrome, carcinoma of endometrium. In obese and leanness related individuals it may present with non-alcholic fatty liver disease (NAFLD) and sleep apnea.

There is considerable heterogeneity in the clinical findings, and variation in the same patient over time. Acne is less of a marker of PCOS as compared to hirsutism. Hirsutism and acanthosis nigricans are the most reliable cutaneous markers of PCOS. Their presence should raise clinical concern and warrant further diagnostic evaluation.

As per ESHRE/ASRM-sponsored third PCOS consensus workshop group: Acne and androgenic alopecia are prevalent but unreliable markers of biochemical hyperandrogenism. Acne is not commonly associated with hyperandrogenemia, and should not be regarded as evidence of hyperandrogenemia.[7]

Acne Presentation in PCOS

Acne in PCOS is usually of moderate to severe grade. Inflammatory lesions predominate on lower face, neck (facial V area), chest and upper back. It begins or persists into adulthood (over the age of 25 years) and flares severely with menstrual cycle. It is usually resistant to conventional therapy and relapses shortly even after isotretinoin therapy.[8]

Phenotypes of PCOS

Based on clinical features and laboratory investigations, there are different phenotypes of PCOS and includes following (Table 6.2):

- Ovulatory PCOS (HA + PCOM).
- Classic PCOS Type 1 (OM + HA + PCOM).
- Normoandrogenic PCOS (OM + PCOM).
- Classic PCOS Type 2 [NIH PCOS] (OM + HA).

Following factors are important for deciding further investigations.[9]

Biochemical Characteristics

High BMI for overweight/obesity >23 kg/m^2 for adults and >97.5th percentile for age in adolescents.

Insulin resistance (acanthosis nigricans as clinical marker of insulin resistance).

Family history of diabetes or PCOS, obesity and any marker of lipid metabolic dysregulation (elevated serum total cholesterol, triglyceride and LDL-C and HDL levels).

Clinical symptoms mainly include pubertal deviations in terms of early or late, disturbances in periodicity and timing of menstrual cycle, presence of PCO and clinical signs of hyperandrogenism such as early acne or hirsutism, persistent severe acne, frequent relapse in acne, acne in facial 'V' area, and hirsutism for more than two years.

Diagnostic Criteria for PCOS (Box 6.1)

A recent National Institute of Health (NIH)-sponsored workshop on PCOS endorsed the Rotterdam criteria for diagnosis of PCOS.

Diagnosis of PCOS as per Rotterdam criteria at least 2 of the following 3.

Firstly, irregular cycles/anovulation which includes either oligomenorrhea (OM), that is, <8 (6–9) cycles per year or >35 days cycle and secondly amenorrhea.

Thirdly, hyperandrogenism (HA), clinically defined as hirsutism and acne, and involves biochemical tests like testosterone—total, free and free androgen index is raised.

Table 6.2: Phenotypes of PCOS

	Type I classic PCOS (A, HA, PCO)	*Type II classic (A, HA)*	*Ovulatory PCOS (HA, PCO)*	*Normoandrogenic or mild PCOS (A, PCO, ±HA)*
Menstrual cycle	Irregular	Irregular	Normal	Irregular
Ultrasound	Polycystic	Normal	Polycystic	Polycystic
Serum androgens	High	High	High	Normal or slightly elevated
Hirsutism	+	+	+	–
Obesity	+	+	+	–
Insulin resistance	Present	Present	Present	Not present
Long-term sequelae	Potential long-term	Potential long-term	Unknown	Unknown
Prevalence	53–61%	7–8.9%	16–29%	8–16%

A: Anovulation; *HA:* Hyperandrogenism; *PCO:* Polycystic ovary.

Box 6.1: Criteria for the definition of polycystic ovary syndrome (PCOS)

NIH statement (1990)

To include all of the following:

1. Hyperandrogenism and/or hyperandrogenemia
2. Oligo-ovulation
3. Exclusion of related disorders*

ESHRE/ASRM statement (Rotterdam, 2003)

To include two of the following, in addition to exclusion of related disorders:*

1. Oligo-ovulation or anovulation (e.g. amenorrhea, irregular uterine bleeding)
2. Clinical and/or biochemical signs of hyperandrogenism (e.g. hirsutism, elevated serum total or free testosterone)
3. Polycystic ovaries (by ultrasonography)

AES suggested criteria for the diagnosis of PCOS (2006)

To include all of the following:

1. *Hyperandrogenism:* Hirsutism and/or hyperandrogenemia
2. *Ovarian dysfunction:* Oligo-anovulation and/or polycystic ovaries
3. Exclusion of other androgen excess of related disorders*

*Includes ruling out other disorders

Polycystic ovarian morphology (PCOM) by ultrasound shows following findings:

a. Ovarian volume >10 ml and/or
b. >12 follicles (now > = 25 with high resolution devices, transducer frequency > = 8 MHz) in each ovary measuring 2–9 mm in diameter on day 2–5 of menses, post-menstrual in adolescents
c. Only one ovary fitting this definition is sufficient.

Rotterdam criteria/exclusion criteria include ruling out the other disorders like adrenal excess—non-classical congenital adrenal hyperplasia (NC-CAH) laboratory tests include: 17α-HP (hydroxyprogesterone), DHEAS and thyroid dysfunction, serum free T3, T4, TSH, serum prolactin (more than 20 ng/ml).

Tumors with high serum levels, and with signs of virilisation include Cushing's syndrome and drug induced androgen excess and syndromes associated with insulin resistance.

List of biochemical investigations for diagnosis of PCOS includes:

1. Free T3, T4, TSH. Hypothyroidism: If TSH upper limit (0.5 μIU/ml. Hyperthyroidism: If TSH lower limit (0.1 μIU/ml).

2. Prolactin: > Upper limit of normal (2–29 ng/ml).
3. Proving biochemical hyperandrogenism is usually difficult and is mainly done on day 2–5 of menstrual cycle, 8 am fasting sample and in women whose cycles are irregular or > 45 days—may be done at any point of time.
4. Direct free testosterone: Clinician should be aware of the limitations of measurements performed without rigorous quality control.

List of biochemical investigations for diagnosis of hyperinsulinemia and metabolic syndrome summates BMI, waist to hip ratio, blood pressure, serum fasting and post-prandial insulin, insulin resistance (IR) which is fasting glucose/ fasting insulin and value of <4.5 is suggestive of IR and serum lipid profile.

Anti-müllerian hormone (AMH), as a surrogate to (absence of) USG, is under consideration. Its cut-off values vary with ethnicity. Though, it is useful, in the absence of standardized assay techniques and accepted cut-off levels in all ethnicities, results for diagnosis of PCOS are to be interpreted with caution.

CONGENITAL ADRENAL HYPERPLASIA

It comprises a group of autosomal-recessively inherited disorders caused by defect in biosynthetic pathway of cortisol and/or aldosterone.

Enzyme defects cause glucocorticoid deficiency and an overproduction of biosynthetic precursor steroids.

Adrenal androgen biosynthesis is not impaired—a massive reactive overproduction due to increased ACTH secretion within the upregulated hypothalamo-pituitary- adrenal system.

95% cases are due to 21-hydroxylase deficiency, caused by inactivating mutations in the 21-hydroxylase gene (CYP21A2). Different CYP21 mutations result in varying degrees of impaired 21-OH activity and cause a spectrum of disease expression.

NON-CLASSIC CONGENITAL ADRENAL HYPERPLASIA (NCCAH)

It is a milder, late-onset form with partial impairment of 21-OH activity which affects 1% of the general population, while many patients may remain undiagnosed. It is reported in 1.2–30% of hirsute, oligomenorrheic women. Acne is a prominent finding in women with NC-CAH which persists from peripubertal period to adult life.

In men acne may be the only symptom of androgen excess—reports of male acne patients in whom hormonal screening revealed irregularities suggestive of late-onset CAH.

Diagnosis for NCCAH

- 17-hydroxyprogesterone
- <2 ng/dl is normal
- >8 ng/ml is diagnostic of late onset CAH
- 2–8 ng/ml necessitates ACTH stimulated 17-hydroxy-progesterone assay
- MRI of abdomen since adrenals are not visualized on USG to rule out other causes.

SAHA SYNDROME

Presence of seborrhea, acne, hirsutism and alopecia in women—first summarized as SAHA syndrome in 1982.

All four major signs are present in approximately 20% of patients.

Seborrhea always present, acne occurs in 10%, androgenetic alopecia in 21%, and hirsutism in 6%. It generally occurs in young to middle-aged women and involves hyperandrogenism, either presence of elevated blood levels of androgens or increased androgen-driven peripheral response with normal circulating androgen levels.

In males—patterned alopecia, AN and acne.

APAAN (acne, patterned alopecia, acanthosis nigricans) syndrome is the term suggested for this presentation. Acne in men is related to insulin resistance, and higher degrees are more consistently linked with IR and found in severe acne. Association with metabolic syndrome not statistically significant.

HAIR-AN

HAIR-AN is characterized by coexistence of: Hyperandrogenism (HA), insulin resistance (IR) and acanthosis nigricans

(AN) which is considered as a unique subtype of PCOS and impaired glucose tolerance. Five percent of women with hyperandrogenemia, are considered to have this condition.

Its clinical presentation includes symptoms which are resultant of increased androgens and insulin levels. Clinical signs show hyperandrogenemia, such as seborrhea, acne, hirsutism, menstrual irregularities, androgenic alopecia, deepening of voice, clitoromegaly, and changes in muscle mass. IR with diabetic symptoms as well as AN. Accompanying findings are obesity, hyperglycemia, hyperlipidemia, infertility.

Biochemical parameters in HAIR-AN has markedly elevated insulin levels, elevated or high-normal levels of testosterone and androstenedione, normal levels of luteinizing hormone and prolactin. Adrenal function is usually normal.

AUTOINFLAMMATORY CONDITIONS: IL-1 ABNORMALITIES

Autoinflammatory syndromes and acne include SAPHO, PAPA, PASH, and PAPASH syndromes that share the manifestations of joint disease and severe acne. Alterations in innate immunity, autoimmunity, adaptive immunity, and autoinflammation have been proposed in causation of this syndromes. It is characterized by inflammasomes activation leading to release of proinflammatory interleukin-1 (IL-1). *Propionibacterium acnes* further activates inflammasomes in the skin leading to IL-1 release.

Pathophysiology of autoinflammatory syndromes suggest over-activation of innate immune system leading to increased production of the interleukin-1 (IL-1) family and 'sterile' neutrophil-rich cutaneous inflammation with over- expression tumor necrosis factor-α (TNF-α).

Management includes biological drugs specifically targeting these cytokines.

SAPHO Syndrome

It is an acronym for synovitis, acne, pustulosis, hyperostosis, and osteitis. It is a rare chronic disease involving skin, bone, and joints.

Osteoarticular symptoms vary from slight to severe pain, with or without swelling. Affected bones include chest wall (sternocostal, sternoclavicular, and manubriosternal joint), sacroiliac joints, spine, and extremities. High fever and weight loss also often present.

Variable skin findings include palmoplantar pustulosis (55%) which is most common skin manifestation, acne (25%), including acne conglobata, acne fulminans, and HS-less frequently associated.

Diagnosis will include skin biopsy which shows neutrophilic infiltration. Other tools are MRI, CT, etc.

PAPA Syndrome

The clinical triad of pyogenic sterile arthritis, pyoderma gangrenosum (PG) and acne conglobata was noted in several families and described with the acronym PAPA syndrome in 1997.[10] In 2002, the gene of CD2-binding protein 1 (CD2BP1; also called proline/serine/threonine phosphatase-interacting protein1, PSTPIP1) on chromosome 15q24–25.1 was identified as the gene causing the syndrome.[11,12]

The CD2BP1 protein binds pyrin, which is an inhibitor of the inflammatory process. In PAPA syndrome, the mutated CD2BP1 protein has enhanced binding capacity to pyrin and prevents the bound pyrin from acting. As pyrin is expressed on neutrophils, but not on T or B cells, the decreased amount of unbound pyrin results in neutrophilic infiltration in arthritis, acne, PG and other neutrophilic dermatoses.

Mostly, arthritis is the earliest sign occurring between age 1 and 16 years.[13] Being aseptic and seronegative, the pauci-articular, non-axial arthritis of variable severity commonly affects hands, elbows, knees and ankles. Axial joints were involved in a few cases. At puberty, severe nodulocystic acne develops. PG occurs in adolescence or adulthood, usually after the appearance of acne. The transition of PAPA syndrome from inflammatory arthritis to cutaneous manifestation with acne and PG at puberty is notable.

Association of PAPA syndrome with other diseases has been described, such as proteinuria, insulin-dependent diabetes mellitus, hypogammaglobulinemia, idiopathic hepatitis and uveitis.[10] As none of these diseases is uniformly present, the association may merely be a coincidence.

Of the triad, PG and acne may be present for decades. Sterile pyogenic arthritis is generally self-limiting, but prolonged prominent arthritis can lead to joint destruction and deformity.

Apert Syndrome (Acrocephalosyndactyly)

Prevalence is estimated to be 15/1,000,000 making up approximately 4% of all cases of craniosynostosis. It is inherited as autosomal dominant pattern. It is characterized by synostoses of extremities, vertebrae, and skull, with syndactyly of fingers and toes. It often begins in early puberty, characterized by seborrhea and moderate to severe acne with an unusual distribution with lesions extending to forearms.

Histologic examination exhibits dilated follicular infundibula extending to mid-dermis, follicular abscesses in upper and mid-portions of corium, and numerous larger sebaceous lobules.

Plasma androgen levels and androgen receptor staining of sebaceous glands are normal.

Borrone Dermato-Cardio-Skeletal (BDCS) Syndrome

It is a severe progressive autosomal recessive disorder characterized by coarse facies, thick skin, acne conglobata, dysmorphic facies, vertebral abnormalities and mitral valve prolapse. Caused by loss-of-function mutations in SH3PXD2B.[14]

CONCLUSION

Acne is a chronic disease and a reflection of disturbances of hormonal and, at times, immunological milieu. Appropriate hormonal evaluation of all cases of atypical acne is to be done.

An understanding of dermato-endocrinology, in terms of pathogenetic mechanisms of hormonal acne, methodology of hormonal assays and their limitations in the clinical practice needs to be known. In depth knowledge of hormonal interventions enables to design a treatment road map that will optimize results of acne associated with systemic disease.

REFERENCES

1. Majumdar A. Comparison of clinical features and health manifestations in lean vs. obese Indian women with PCOS. J Hum Reprod Sci 2009;2:12–7.
2. Zouboulis CC. [Acne vulgaris. The role of hormones]. Hautarzt. 2010 Feb;61(2):107–8, 110–4.
3. Jayakar Thomas, Kumar Parimalam, Ragavi B Sindhu. Hormonal Acne: Leading to a Paradigm Shift in the Management of Acne. Expert Rev Dermatol. 2013;8(3):225–7.
4. Madnani et al. Indian J Dermatol Venereol Leprol 2013;79:310–21.
5. Zoubolis CC. Acne as a chronic systemic disease. Clin Dermatol. 2014 May-Jun;32(3):389–96.
6. Cedars MI. Cutaneous Findings and Systemic Associations in Women With Polycystic Ovary Syndrome. JAMA Dermatol. 2016 Apr;152(4):391–8.
7. Consensus on women's health aspects of polycystic ovary syndrome (PCOS): the Amsterdam ESHRE/ASRM-Sponsored 3rd PCOS Consensus Workshop Group. 2012 Jan;97(1):28–38.e25.
8. Trivedi MK, Shinkai K, A Review of hormone-based therapies to treat adult acne vulgaris in women. 2017 Mar 30;3(1):44–52.
9. Malik et al. A Consensus Evidence-based Good Clinical Practice Recommendations. Fertility Science and Research/Jan- Jun 2014, Vol 1, Issue 1.
10. Lindor NM, Arsenault TM, Solomon H et al. A new autosomal dominant disorder of pyogenic sterile arthritis, pyoderma gangrenosum,and acne: Papa syndrome. Mayo Clin Proc 1997;72:611–615.
11. Wise CA, Gillum JD, Seidman CE et al. Mutations in CD2BP1 disrupt binding to PTP PEST and are responsible for PAPA syndrome, an autoinflammatory disorder. Hum Mol Genet 2002;11:961–969.
12. Kanazawa N, Furukawa F. Autoinflammatory syndromes with a dermatological perspective. J Dermatol 2007;34:601–618.
13. Stichweh DS, Punaro M, Pascual V. Dramatic improvement of pyoderma gangrenosum with infliximab in a patient with papa syndrome. Pediatr Dermatol 2005;22:262–265.
14. Wilson GR, Sunley J, Smith KR, Pope K, Bromhead CJ, Fitzpatrick E, Di Rocco M, Van Steensel M, Coman DJ, Leventer RJ, Delatycki MB. Mutations in SH3PXD2B cause Borrone dermato-cardio-skeletal syndrome. European Journal of Human Genetics. 2014 Jun;22(6):741–7.

CHAPTER 7

Clinical Variants

A number of variants of acne are recognized as follows:
1. Severe forms (acne fulminans and acne conglobata).
2. Drug-induced.
3. Cosmetic acne.
4. Occupational acne.
5. Acne associated with psychological problems: Acne excoriee.
6. Acne mechanica.
7. Pre-pubertal acne.
8. Post-adolescent acne.

ACNE FULMINANS

Introduction

Acne fulminans is a severe destructive form of acne with acute onset and systemic symptoms occurring mainly in adolescent males and affects primarily the trunk and the face.

Synonym

- Acne maligna.
- Acute febrile ulcerative acne conglobate.[1]

Associated Diseases

SAPHO syndrome has been found to be associated with acne fulminans. This has been attributed to systemic inflammatory cytokinemia. The successful treatment of acne fulminans associated with SAPHO syndrome by infliximab supports this hypothesis.[2]

Acne fulminans associated with Crohn's disease has also been reported.[3]

PAPA syndrome can be associated with both acne fulminans and acne conglobata.

Pathophysiology

Various factors like infection, genetic susceptibility or autoimmune factors have been suggested. Response to systemic corticosteroids, increase in globulins and decreased levels of complement point towards an autoimmune etiology. Defective innate immunity (IL-1 pathway) has also been suggested. Isotretinoin therapy might trigger AF in patients with severe acne, particularly when treatment is initiated at high doses. This form of the disease does not usually have systemic symptoms.[1]

Clinical Features

Patients typically present with a history of mild to moderate acne for a mean of 2 years followed by acute onset of ulcerative and necrotic acne along with fever, arthralgia and other systemic symptoms (Fig. 7.1). Typically they do not respond to systemic antibacterials (Table 7.1).

The lesions are numerous, inflammatory, tender and ulcerative nodules covered with hemorrhagic crusts mainly over the upper chest, back, shoulders and even the face and pyogenic granuloma-like lesions may be present.

Systemic signs and symptoms like malaise, arthralgia, joint swellings, myalgia, fever, anorexia and weight loss are present.

Complete blood count shows marked leucocytosis which may be leukemoid.

Bone involvement in the form of lytic lesions is common.

Differential Diagnosis

Severe acne conglobata can closely mimic acne fulminans but a gradual onset, lack of systemic symptoms and presence of double comedones can differentiate it from acne fulminans.

Complications

Significant and disfiguring scarring is the most common complication. Other complications are mild musculoskeletal discomfort and radiological changes like hyperostosis and sclerosis.

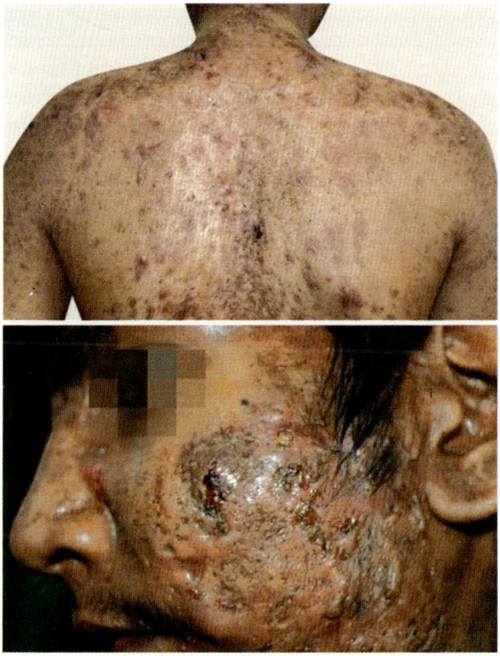

Fig. 7.1: Multiple noduloulcerative and necrotic lesions present over face and trunk (Acne fulminans)

Table 7.1: Terminology of acne fulminans[1]	
Acne fulminans with systemic symptoms (AF-SS)	Abrupt, flare of acne, with erosions with crusts, ulcers, hemorrhagic nodules/plaques. Systemic findings like -fever, malaise, bone pain, arthralgias, erythema nodosum, and leukocytosis. Laboratory abnormalities may include anemia, leukocytosis, elevated ESR, and CRP X-ray findings: Osteolytic bony lesions; usually at sternum, clavicles, sacroiliac joints, hips
Acne fulminans without systemic symptoms (AF-WOSS)	Acute flare of inflammatory acne, with erosions with crusts, ulcers, and hemorrhagic nodules/ plaques without systemic findings
Isotretinoin induced acne fulminans with systemic symptoms (IIAFWSS)	Drug-induced form of acne fulminans with systemic symptoms (rarely it can be caused by testosterone and anabolic steroids; this condition is much less common than IIAF-WOSS)

(Contd.)

Table 7.1: Terminology of acne fulminans[1] (*contd.*)	
Isotretinoin induced acne fulminans without systemic symptoms (IIAFWOSS)	Drug-induced form of acne fulminans without systemic symptoms (other drugs including testosterone and anabolic steroids can cause IIAF-WOSS; this condition is the most common form of AF)

Management

First Line Therapy

Oral prednisolone 0.5–1.0 mg/kg/day should be started and tapered slowly over 2–3 months. Low dose oral isotretinoin (0.25–0.5 mg/kg/day) is then cautiously introduced after active inflammation subsides, i.e. usually after 3–4 weeks of either systemic steroid therapy as isotretinoin has been reported to paradoxically cause acne fulminans in some patients.[4]

Alternative Therapies

Clofazimine 200 mg three times a week has been shown to improve acne fulminans.

Isotretinoin in combination with dapsone has been used successfully to treat acne fulminans associated with erythema nodosum.

Biologics especially TNF-inhibitors have been shown to be effective especially acne fulminans associated with auto-inflammatory disease.[13]

Cases that have not been responding to Isotretinoin are successfully treated with IL-1 inhibitors (e.g. anakinra) as well as immunosuppressive agents like Azathioprine and Cyclosporine.[1]

NSAIDs and graduated physical exercise helps to treat fever and joint pains.

ACNE CONGLOBATA

Introduction

Acne conglobata is a severe form of acne characterized by multiple inflammatory papules, tender nodules, abscesses and malodorous draining sinuses and tracts (Fig. 7.2). Multiple

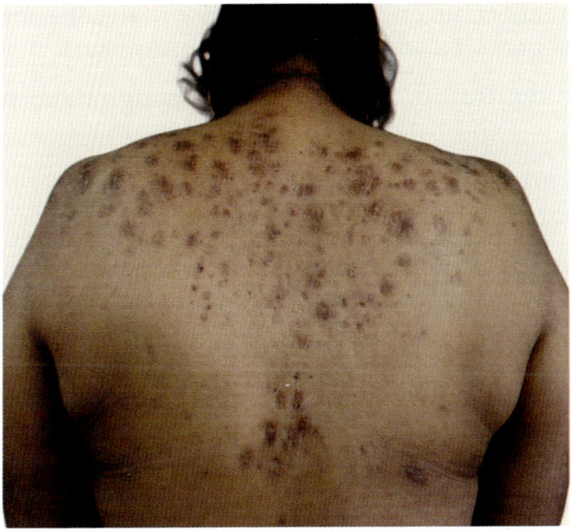

Fig. 7.2: Multiple papules, nodules and comedones present over back (Acne conglobata)

polyporous, grouped comedones are typical and extensive disfiguring hypertrophic and atrophic scars are also common features.

It may occur in the setting of existing papulo-pustular acne or may present as a relapse of acne that has been in remission for many years. The onset of lesions is relatively gradual with absence of systemic symptoms as opposed to acne fulminans. The lesions commonly occur on the trunk and upper limbs but also extend to the buttocks (Fig. 7.2). The malodorous, discharging sinus tracts and significant scarring frequently result in psychological impairment.

Epidemiology

Age and Sex

Acne conglobata has a male preponderance and usually presents in the third or fourth decade.

Associations

It is usually a part of follicular occlusion triad, i.e. dissecting cellulitis of scalp, hidradenitis suppurativa, acne conglobata.

Follicular occlusion tetrad adds pilonidal sinus and follicular occlusion pentad adds epidermal inclusion cyst.[5]

SAPHO syndrome: Synovitis, acne conglobata, pustulosis, hyperostosis and osteitis.[2]

PAPA syndrome: Severe acne conglobata with sterile pyogenic arthritis and pyoderma gangrenosum.

PASH syndrome: Triad of pyoderma gangrenosum, acne conglobata and suppurative hidradenitis.

PASS syndrome: Includes pyoderma gangrenosum, acne conglobata, suppurative hidradenitis and seronegative spondyloarthritis.[6]

MARSH syndrome: Melasma, acne, rosacea, seborrhoeic eczema and hirsutism.[7]

Pathophysiology

The primary cause of acne conglobata remains unknown. Various predisposing factors like anabolic steroid abuse, increased testosterone or testosterone withdrawal or any androgen secreting tumor and even exposure to halogenated aromatic hydrocarbons are implicated.

Genetics

Familial cases have been reported with linkage to chromosome 15q24–26 in the region of IL-16 and CRABP1 genes.

PAPA syndrome is caused by mutations in the gene on chromosome 15 that encodes proline-serine-threonine phosphatase interacting protein 1 (PSTPIP1; also known as CD2 antigen-binding protein 1 [CD2BP1]).[8]

Clinical Features

Acne conglobata may develop in the setting of acne vulgaris that has been quiescent for a number of years but frequently the onset is insidious with a chronic. It is more common in males.

Patients present with multiple comedones, inflammatory papulo-pustules, nodules, abscesses and interconnecting sinuses (Fig. 7.2). Patients may also have atrophic and hypertrophic scars.

Management

Oral isotretinoin (0.5–1 mg/kg/day) for 4–6 months is the first line of treatment.

To control the inflammation, prednisolone 1 mg/kg/day for 2–4 weeks can be combined with isotretinoin.[7]

Surgical management is done for abscesses and sinuses. Tetracyclines and dapsone form the second line treatment so as to decrease inflammation.

DRUG-INDUCED ACNE

It can occur as a side-effect of many oral or topical drugs. Patients typically present with an abrupt onset of monomorphous papulopustules usually over the back, arms and shoulders. This feature differentiates drug-induced acne from other acne variants.

Most common drug implicated is oral corticosteroids. Topical application of corticosteroids leads to development of monomorphic acne lesions over erythematous base. Lesions usually subside after the drug is stopped but at times it leads to prolonged or severe flares after withdrawal of the drug.

Other common drugs causing drug-induced acne are as follows:

- Anabolic steroids (danazol, testosterone)[14]
- Corticotropin
- EGFR inhibitors
- Progestins
- Antidepressants: Lithium, amoxapine
- Anticonvulsants: Carbamazepine, phenytoin, pheno- barbital
- Barbiturates
- DHEA
- Halogens: Iodide, chloride, bromide, halothane
- Antitubercular drugs: Isoniazid, rifampicin
- Cyclosporine
- Vitamins B_{12}, B_6, cyanocobalamin
- TNF-α inhibitors
- Azathioprine

ACNE VENETATA

Venerium is latin word means poison. In this context it means poisonous for sebaceous follicles. It is a contact acne. Occurs due to epicutaneous contact. Rarer route of contacts are by inhalation (e.g. chloracne) or ingestion.[9] It includes following variants.

Acne Cosmetica

It occurs due to long-term use of cosmetics containing comedogenic substances like lanolin, petrolatum, certain vegetable oils, butyl stearate, lauryl alcohol and oleic acid.

Patients present with predominantly comedonal acne mainly closed comedones.

Pomade Acne

Pomade is a greasy, waxy, or a water-based substance that is used to style hair.

Pomade acne is a subtype of acne vulgaris induced when pomades and other oil-based grooming substances that have been applied to the scalp migrate onto facial skin.

It presents as closed comedones on the forehead and temple. The cheeks and chin may also be involved if the offending agent was applied to the entire face.

Occupational Acne

Occupational acne occurs after exposure to insoluble, follicle-occluding substances at the workplace.

Substances commonly responsible are cutting oils, petroleum-based products, chlorinated aromatic hydrocarbons, and coal tar derivatives. People who work with electrical conductors and insulators, fungicides, pesticides, wood preservatives and herbicides are prone to develop occupational acne.[10]

Clinical Features

It presents mainly with comedones, varying numbers of papules, pustules and cystic lesions distributed on exposed as well as typically covered areas.

Oil and Tar Acne

It occurs in regions that come in contact with oil and tar products. Men are more affected than females.

Occurs within 6 weeks of exposure to oil and tar over exposed as well as covered areas of the body.

Lower arms and thighs are commonly involved.

In patients of acne vulgaris, there is increased tendency of development of occupational acne than in non-acne prone patients.

The commonest oils involved are the impure paraffin mixtures used in the engineering industry and petroleum products, coal-tar distillates, especially pitch and creosote.

Chloracne ("Madish"—Metabolising Acquired Dioxin Induced Skin Hamartomas)[11]

It occurs after exposure to chlorinated aromatic hydrocarbons. Lesions are usually located on both sides of the head and neck, especially on the temporal, retroauricular and mandibular regions but in more severe cases the chloracne may occur on other parts of the body including the axillae, scrotum, extremities, trunk and buttocks.

Multiple comedones with inflammatory papules and pustules are seen along with pigmentation, hypertrichosis and palmar and plantar hyperhidrosis.

Ophthalmic chloracne may occur, due to the meibomian gland involvement.

Systemic abnormalities are less frequent but when present include fatigue, anorexia, neuropathy, impotence, disturbed liver function and hyperlipidaemia.

The chloracne and systemic disturbances may last for many years following exposure.

Treatment

Topical therapy with retinoids such as adapalene sand tretinoin are worthy of a therapeutic trial; long-term oral antibiotic therapy may be needed for the inflammatory lesions.

Oral isotretinoin does not help since the sebaceous gland has already undergone atrophy.

Gentle cautery under local anaesthetic cream (EMLA® applied for 60–75 min under polythene occlusion) produces excellent results. Litigation is frequent when the contamination follows an industrial accident.

ACNE AESTIVALIS

Also known as 'Acne Mallorca', 'Tropical acne'. It is type of polymorphous light eruption induced by ultra violet A radiation. It is seasonal, usually affecting people in springtime. Usually present with mono-morphous eruption that consists of multiple, uniform, red, papular lesions. It is delayed-type hypersensitivity reaction. Onset is 24–72 hours after sun exposure.[12]

ACNE MECHANICA

Acne mechanica occurs due to obstruction of pilosebaceous duct leading to comedo formation due to repeated rubbing or friction. For example, rubbing by helmets, chin straps and collars or fiddler's neck, which occurs due to repetitive friction from violin placement on the neck. It presents as a lichenified, hyperpigmented plaque with comedones.

Treatment is aimed at eliminating the causative friction.

PREADOLESCENT ACNE

Definition

It is an uncommon variant of acne that occurs before puberty. Classification of acne in children based on age includes five subtypes:

1. Neonatal
2. Infantile
3. Mid-childhood
4. Pre-adolescent, and
5. Adolescent

Introduction

Prepubertal acne has numerous presentations and thus it is sometimes misdiagnosed.

It can help in identification of children who are at risk of virilization. Complete clinical examination and careful history taking is necessary for early diagnosis and treatment of hormonal abnormalities, adrenal and gonadal tumours.

Age and Gender

Neonatal acne: A neonate is defined as a newborn up to 35 days of age. Neonatal acne presents at birth to the age of 4–6 weeks and is seen more frequently in boys (5:1) (Fig. 7.3).

Infantile acne: Typically presents between 3 and 12 months but may occur as late as 16 months. It is more common in boys.

Mid-childhood acne: It occurs between age of 1 and 7 years.

Pre-pubertal acne: Presents before true puberty.

Adrenarche represents maturation of the adrenal glands with adrenal production of hormones and development of the zona reticularis and acquisition of enzymes that facilitate synthesis of androgens from cholesterol. Adrenarche occurs at the age of 6–7 years in girls and 7–8 years in boys.

Prepubertal acne may occur from age 7 to 11 years.

Pathophysiology

Development of prepubertal acne is directly related to hyperactivity of the sebaceous glands which are stimulated by neonatal androgens from the testes in boys and adrenals in girls and boys. Maternal androgens can be transferred transplacentally and the hyperactive neonatal adrenal glands in both sexes result in an increased production of DHEA and its sulphated form, i.e. DHEAS. During the neonatal period and for approximately 1 year afterwards, the adrenals secrete androgens. This androgen production also increases again in mid-childhood around 7 years of age. Ultimately, it causes hypersecretion of sebum and development of acne.

An inflammatory response to *Malassezia* spp. (e.g. sympodialis, furfur) has also been proposed as the etiology of neonatal acne. This is further supported by effective treatment with topical imidazoles (2% ketoconazole cream).

Clinical Features

1. **Neonatal acne:** It presents as erythematous papulo- pustular lesions commonly distributed on the cheeks, face and forehead (Fig. 7.3).

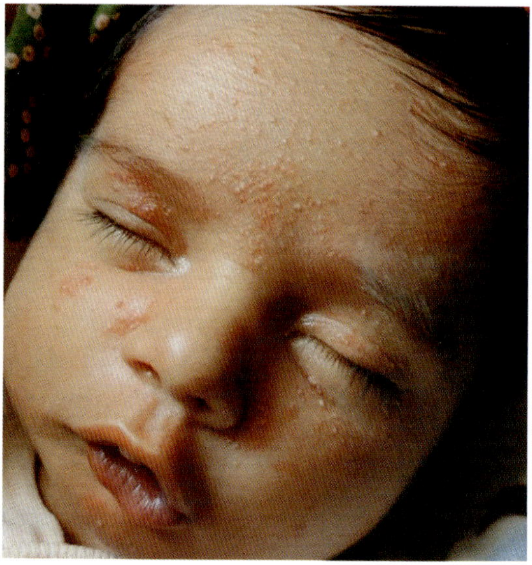

Fig. 7.3: Neonatal acne

2. **Infantile acne:** Inflamed papule and pustule with open and closed comedones diffusely involving the entire cheeks.
3. **Mid-childhood acne:** Acne at this age always need to rule out androgen access.
4. **Pre-adolescent and adolescent acne:** Presents as centrofacial comedonal lesions and early onset of significant numbers of comedones is predictive of the development of severe, inflammatory acne as a teenager.

Disease Course and Prognosis

Neonatal acne resolves spontaneously with a little scarring.

Infantile acne has long and variable duration and course, resolves up to five years of age and scarring occurs if deep seated lesions.

Treatment

Neonatal acne is benign and transient. Parents need to be reassured.

Topical imidazole cream can be prescribed.

POST-ADOLESCENT ACNE

Acne persisting or occurring for the first time after 25 years of age in females (Table 7.2).

Usually there is history of premenstrual flare.

They present as tender deep-seated papulo-nodules along the jawline and neck.

Hyperandrogenism is found in one-third of these women and hormonal therapy is effective.

ACNE EXCORIEE

Acne excoriee is regarded as repetitive and compulsive picking of the skin lesions predominantly on the face (Fig. 7.4).

Underlying psychological problem may include obsessive compulsive disorder, tension, anxiety or stress.

Clinically, it is characterized by linear excoriation marks, inflammatory papules with a few crusted lesions resulting in a lot of PIH (Fig. 7.5) and even scarring.

Treatment

Cognitive behavioral therapy with habit reversal techniques is useful. Some patients only need to stop the picking habit.

Table 7.2: Differences between adolescent and adult acne

	Adolescent acne	*Adult acne*
Age	Puberty and adolescence	>25 years
Sex	More common in males	Predominantly in females
Severity	Varying from mild comedonal to severe nodulocystic	Commonly low grade inflammatory, popular
Predominant type of lesion	Comedones	Inflammatory papulo-pustules
Sebum production	Increased	Normal or increased
Microbial flora	*P. acnes*	*P. acnes*
Hormonal influences	May occur	More common
Response to treatment	Expected outcome	Often resistant

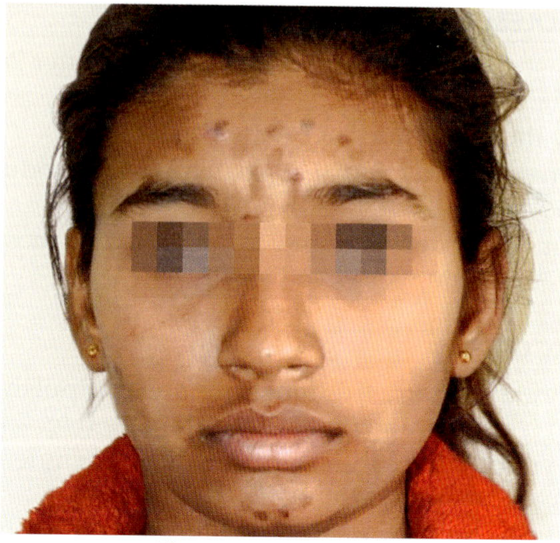

Fig. 7.4: Acne excoriee

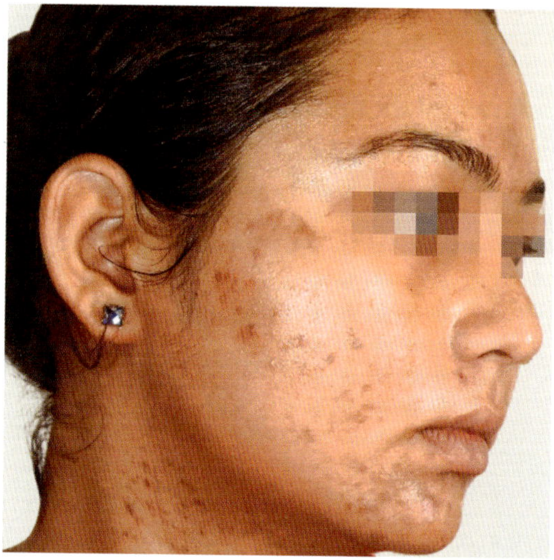

Fig. 7.5: Post-inflammatory hyperpigmentation due to acne

It can be combined with psychotropic drug therapy.

Selective serotonin reuptake inhibitors including fluoxetine, paroxetine, sertraline and fluvoxamine are treatments of choice and are frequently employed alongside psychotherapy.

REFERENCES

1. Greywal T, Zaenglein AL, Baldwin HE, Bhatia N, Chernoff KA, Del Rosso JQ, Eichenfield LF, Levin MH, Leyden JJ, Thiboutot DM, Webster GF. Evidence-based recommendations for the management of acne fulminans and its variants. Journal of the American Academy of Dermatology. 2017 Jul 1;77(1):109–17.
2. Iqbal M, Kolodney MS. Acne fulminans and synovitis acne pustulosis hyperostosis osteitis (SAPHO) syndrome treated with infliximab. J Am Acad Dermatol 2005;52 (5 Suppl. 1):S118– 20.2.
3. Kurokawa S, Tokura Y, Nham NX, et al. Acne fulminans coexisting with pyoderma Gangrenosum like eruptions and posterior scleritis. J Dermatol 1996;23:37–41.
4. Allison MA, Dunn CL, Pearson CA. Acne fulminans treated with isotretinoin and pulsed corticosteroid. Pediatr Dermatol 1997;4:39–42.
5. Vasanth V, Chandrashekar BS. Follicular occlusion tetrad. Indian Dermatol Online J. 2014 Oct;5(4):491-3. doi: 10.4103/2229-5178.142517. PMID: 25396138; PMCID: PMC4228650.
6. Yeon HB, Lindon NM, Seidman JG, et al. Pyogenic arthritis, pyoderma gangrenosum and acne syndrome maps to chromosome 15q. Am J Hum Genet 2000;66:1443–8.
7. Griffiths WA. The red face-an overview and delineation of the MARSH syndrome. Clin Exp Dermatol. 1999 Jan;24(1):42-7. doi: 10.1046/j.1365-2230.1999.00406.x. PMID: 10233649.
8. Wise CA, Gillum JD, Seideman CE, et al. Mutations in CD2BP1 disrupt binding to PTP PEST and are responsible for PAPA syndrome, an autoinflammatory disorder. Hum Mol Genet. 2002;11:961–9.
9. Plewig G, Kligman AM. Acne Venenata. In: ACNE and ROSACEA. Springer, Berlin, Heidelberg (2000). https://doi.org/10.1007/978-3-642-59715-2_38.
10. McDonnell JK, Taylor JS. Occupational and environmental acne. In: Kanerva L, Elsner P, Wahlberg JE, Maibach HI, (eds). Handbook of Occupational Dermatology. Berlin: Springer Verlag, 2000:225–33.
11. Schlessinger DI, Robinson CA, Schlessinger J. Chloracne. [Updated 2022 Oct 17]. In: StatPearls [Internet]. Treasure Island (FL): StatPearls Publishing; 2024 Jan.
12. Plewig G, Kligman AM, Plewig G, Kligman AM. Acne Aestivalis (Mallorca Acne). Acne: Morphogenesis and Treatment. 1975:257–9.
13. Campione E, Mazzotta AM, Bianchi L, et al. Severe acne successfully treated with etanercept. Acta Derm Venereol (Stockh) 2006;86:256–7.
14. Melnik B, Jansen T, Grabbe S. Abuse of anabolic androgenic steroids and body building acne: an underestimated health problem. J Dtsch Dermatol Ges 2007;5:110–17.

CHAPTER 8

Acneiform Eruptions

INTRODUCTION

Acneiform eruptions constitute a group of dermatoses that resemble acne vulgaris both in morphology and distribution. Lesions may be papulopustular, nodular or cystic. While acne vulgaris typically consists of comedones, acneiform eruptions usually lack comedones (Table 8.1).

Acne-like eruption develops as a result of infections, hormonal or metabolic abnormalities, genetic disorders, and drug reactions.

DRUG-INDUCED ACNE

The acneiform rashes are inflammatory follicular reactions characterized by erythematous papules and pustules that develop on face, scalp and upper trunk within first month in >90% of patients. It is frequently associated with cosmetic disfigurement, pain, pruritus and secondary infection. Diagnosis is based on the clinical features and history of exposure to a drug known to be causative.

Table 8.1: Difference between acne and acneiform eruptions

Acne	*Acneiform eruptions*
Polymorphic lesions	Monomorphic lesions
Age of onset-usually pubertal	At any age
Gradual onset	Sudden onset
Area of involvement–seborrheic area	Any area involved
Scarring present	Scarring absent

Drug-induced acneiform eruption is to be suspected if the onset of acne is sudden and abrupt in the absence of past history of acne vulgaris. The latency between acne and drug initiation for various types of drugs is different, ranging from shorter latencies seen in systemic corticosteroids and androgens to longer latent period more than 1 month observed with cyclosporine. Median latent period is 7–10 days while maximum severity is seen in the second week.

Drugs Attributed to Acneiform Eruptions

- Steroids (adrenocorticotropic hormone, anabolic steroids like danazol and testosterone, systemic steroids, hormonal contraceptives).
- Antibiotics (mainly antitubercular drugs like isoniazid, rifampicin, ethionamide).
- Halogens (iodides, bromides and chlorides).
- Chemotheraputic agents: Dactinomycin, thiourea, thiouracil.
- Epidermal growth factor receptor inhibitors: Cetuximab.
- Multikinase inhibitors: Imatinib.
- Histone deaetylase inhibitor: Vorinostat
- Neuropsychiatric drugs (tricyclic antidepressants, lithium, valproate, phenytoin, dantrolene)
- JAK-STAT inhibitors (JAK-acne)[11]

  Mechanism of acneiform eruption by JAK inhibitors remains unknown. Possible mechanism could be:
  - JAK-STAT signalling involves downstream signal transduction of epidermal growth factors which leads to follicular hyperkeratinizaton.
  - Immune slant toward Th1 and Th17 and Th2 signalling inhibition.
  - Due to immune inhibition, change in microbiome of skin, including colonization of demodex folliculorum.
- Vitamins B_{12}

  It occurs particularly among adult or elderly females. The onset of these eruptions is acute, occurring days or weeks after the initiation of vitamin B_{12} therapy. Spontaneous and complete remission is commonly observed within a period of 1–8 weeks following the cessation of vitamin B_{12} supplementation, typically occurring within 2–3 weeks.

Recent research indicates that increased levels of vitamin B_{12} in the pilosebaceous follicle can worsen acne. Vitamin B_{12} supplementation in Propionibacterium acnes colonies boosts porphyrin production, leading to skin surface oxidation and the release of pro-inflammatory agents, ultimately promoting the formation of acneiform lesions.[1]

Rarely, eruptions can be caused by vitamins B_1 (thiamine) or B_2 (riboflavin) or B_6 (pyridoxine) supplementation.

Also occurs with following drugs, but uncommon:

- Immunosuppressants (azathioprine, cyclosporine, sirolimus)
- Disulfiram
- Propylthiouracil
- Psoralen + ultraviolet A

STEROIDS

The earliest reports of drug induced adverse effects have been in 1928 when acne-like lesions were described with the use of iodides and chlorinated hydrocarbons. In 1950s, with the introduction of steroids into medical therapy, acneiform eruptions began to be noted as one of their side effects (Fig. 8.1).

Topical and oral preparations that induce or worsen acne include corticosteroids. It is called "steroid acne".

These are characterized by monomorphous dome-shaped papulo-pustules most commonly located on the chest, extremities, with less involvement of the face.

Steroid acne is often encountered in transplant patients, collagen vascular diseases or neurological pathology that requires protracted courses of oral corticosteroids, particularly longer acting ones such as dexamethasone. Topical or inhaled corticosteroids may cause an acneiform eruption of the area of skin under which the topical preparation is applied or in around the nose or mouth in the case of inhaled steroids.

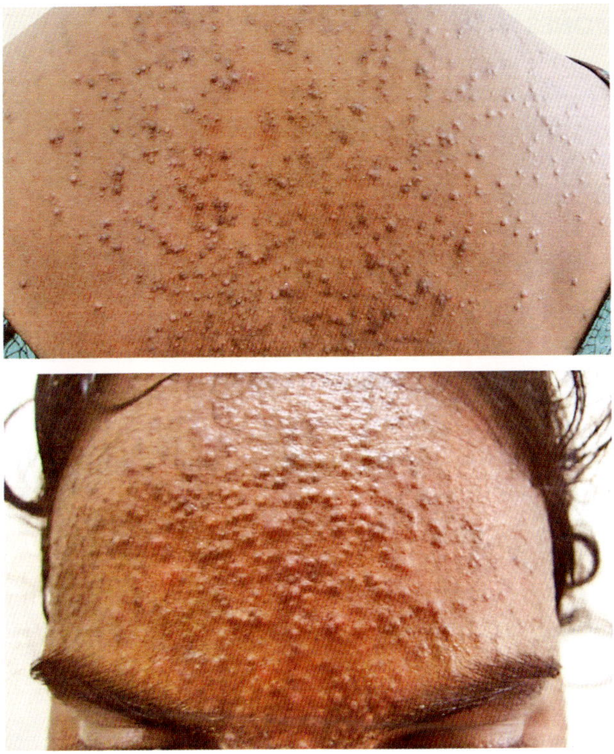

Fig. 8.1: Acneiform eruption due to steroids

Mechanism

It has been suggested that glucocorticoids enhances toll-like receptor-2 expression in human keratinocytes stimulated with *Propionibacterium acnes* or proinflammatory cytokines, resulting in acne.

Histological examination of steroid-induced acne shows local necrosis, follicular plugging and dilatation of hair follicle resulting in an epithelial cyst with intrafollicular and perifollicular neutrophilic inflammatory infiltrate.

Treatment

The eruption usually resolves after discontinuation of the steroid and, in addition, responds to standard treatments of acne vulgaris.

HORMONES

Hormones are a common cause of drug-induced acne. Use of both testosterone and estrogen has been related the development of acne. Body builders who use any type of androgenic or anabolic steroids are at increased risk for developing acne.

A levonorgestrel-releasing intrauterine system (Mirena) has been linked to such new-onset acne.

Calcineurin Inhibitors

There are two types of topical calcineurin inhibitors called tacrolimus (Protopic 0.03% and 0.1%) and pimecrolimus (Elidel). These are classified as immunomodulating agents.

The calcineurin blockers, which affect IL-2 and inhibit T-cell activation and induce local suppression of the adaptive immune system, can cause acne via direct toxicity, chemical modification of sebum or their effect on EGFR and testosterone.

Sirolimus (Rapamune) plus cyclosporine caused in high-risk renal allograft recipients.

Focal acne during topical tacrolimus therapy for vitiligo has been noted.

Cyclosporin

Nodulocystic acne may be induced by the use of cyclosporine in children as well as adults. When it occurs, it can be managed with cessation of cyclosporine therapy and treatment with isotretinoin.

Anticonvulsants

Aromatic anticonvulsant medications have been associated with the induction of acne. This is particularly the case with phenytoin and carbamazepine. An interesting report has linked the development of acne keloidalis in the scalp during treatment with phenytoin and carbamazepine for epilepsy based on the unusual location and clinical presentation and on an *in vitro* mast cell degranulation test.

It is possible that valproate can also be related to new- onset oligomenorrhea with hyperandrogenism and acne.

Psychotropic Medications

Psychotropic medications have been linked to drug-induced acne. Medications as diverse as trazodone and haloperidol have been linked to the development of acne. Aripiprazole which is used to treat schizophrenia, acute manic and mixed episodes associated with bipolar disorder and as an adjunct for the treatment of major depressive disorder has also been a cause of drug-induced acne.

Amineptine, is an atypical tricyclic antidepressant that selectively inhibits the re-uptake of dopamine and, to a lesser extent, norepinephrine. Amineptine, having a powerful and fast-acting antidepressant effect on humans also has a stimulatory and euphoric effect in some patients, has been withdrawn from the market in the United States. Amineptine can result in very severe acneiform eruptions and can be observed in sites not usually affected by acne vulgaris, such as the perineum, arms and legs.

Lithium, which is used to treat bipolar disorders, is a potent inducer of neutrophils and can cause or exacerbate acne. Histologically, in many cases, lithium-induced acne is likely more a form of perifolliculitis with an infiltrate of neutrophils rather than true acne.

Acneiform eruptions tend to occur within the first 6 months of therapy, and they may be linked to lithium's tendency to increase circulating neutrophil chemotaxis, stimulatation of lysosomal enzyme release, and follicular hyperkeratosis.[2]

Epidermal Growth Factor Blockers-PRIDE Complex

Papulopustules and/or paronychia, regulatory abnormalities of hair growth, itching, dryness due to EGFR inhibitors.[3]

National Cancer Institute adverse event scale for acneiform eruptions[4]

- **Grade I:** Intervention not indicated
- **Grade II:** Intervention indicated
- **Grade III:** Associated with pain, disfigurement, ulceration, or desquamation
- **Grade IV:** None
- **Grade V:** Death

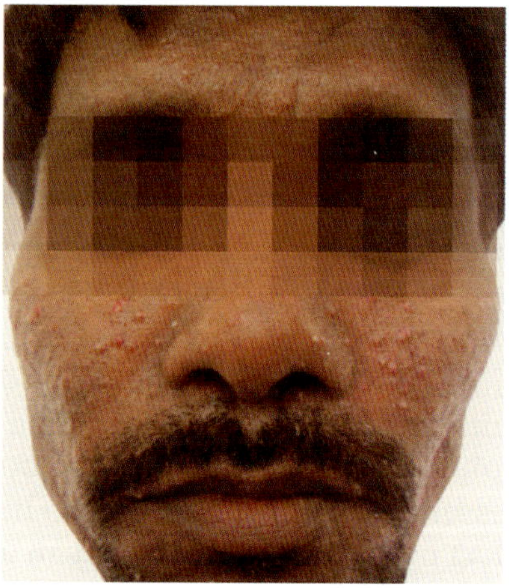

Fig. 8.2: Gefitinib-induced acneiform eruptions

The epidermal growth factor receptor (EGFR) is a transmembrane glycoprotein that is expressed in many normal human cells of epithelial origin, playing an important role in cell growth, differentiation, and proliferation and used for the treatment of advanced lung, pancreatic, colorectal, and head and neck cancers. These include monoclonal antibodies (e.g. cetuximab, panitumumab, necitumumab, pertuzumab) and small-molecule tyrosine kinase inhibitors (e.g. gefitinib, erlotinib, afatinib, osimertinib, lapatinib). The eruption is usually located in the seborrheic areas (rich in sebaceous glands): The face, the neck, the shoulders, the upper trunk (V-shaped), and the scalp (Fig. 8.2).

The acneiform eruption appears a few days after starting treatment with the EGFR inhibitor and reaches a maximum after 2–3 weeks.[5]

Pathogenesis

EGFR is expressed in the basal layer of the epidermis. EGFR inhibitors inhibit both EGFR overexpressed in tumor cells and the one expressed in normal cells of the epidermis. The inhibition of EGFR in keratinocytes induces apoptosis, arrests cell growth, reduces cell migration, and increases cell adhesivity and cell differentiation. All these processes induce keratinocytes to release inflammatory chemokine (CCL2), (CCL5) and (CXCL10).

In particular, the arrest of growth, the migration of keratinocytes, and inflammation cause xerosis and papulopustular acneiform rash.

Epidermal growth factor blockers are linked to an acneiform eruption whose severity parallels clinical effect.

Histologically, two major patterns of reaction have been described:

1. Hyperkeratotic or ectatic follicular infundibula surrounded by a superficial dermal inflammatory cell infiltrate, particularly in the upper portion of the hair follicle, and
2. Neutrophilic suppurative folliculitis with rupture of the epithelial lining.

In particular, cetuximab is commonly linked to an acne-like eruption that is actually like the acneiform eruption of lithium, which is really more of a folliculitis.

Cetuximab does not have to be discontinued if this eruption occurs; it can be treated with topical medications.[6] In fact, some have suggested that an acneiform eruption from cetuximab is indicative of greater therapeutic success. The acne that cetuximab causes does not result in scarring.

OTHER SUBSTANCES THAT MAY INDUCE ACNE

Halogens

They include compounds with chlorides, fluorides and bromides. Chloracne, an acneiform eruption, resulting from blood levels concentration of halogens between 650 and 1200 pg/g. It is most common form of occupational acne.[7]

Pathogenesis

Chloride interferes with vitamin A metabolism in the skin, resulting in disturbances of the epithelial tissues of the pilosebaceous duct.

Chloracne is caused by exposure to certain halogenated polycyclic hydrocarbons such as polychlorinated dibenzodioxins (PCDDs) and dibenzofurans (PCDFs) which are most often found in fungicides, insecticides, herbicides and wood preservatives. It occurs within 2 months of exposure to chloracnegens and can persist for years despite cessation of exposure. The condition is always a sign of systemic exposure to the causal agent, entry may occur via percutaneous absorption as well as from inhalation or ingestion of the chemicals.

Sites of systemic involvement are the eyes, liver and nervous systems.

The iodide-induced eruptions (i.e. iododerma) may be more severe. Patients with bromoderma may also have lesions that resemble pyoderma gangrenosum.

Fluoride in toothpaste has been related to acne-like eruptions. Treatment consists primarily of avoidance of the cause, although topical or oral retinoids are useful. However, chloracne is particularly recalcitrant.

Exogenous Factors that can Cause Acne

Radiation: Radiation-induced acne is rare,[8] clinically and pathogenetically ill-defined acneiform eruption with special features that may occur in irradiated skin areas especially after high doses of deeply penetrating radiation.

It is characterized by comedo-like papules occurring at sites of previous exposure to therapeutic ionizing radiation and disappears as the acute phase of radiation dermatitis starts to resolve.

The ionizing rays induce epithelial metaplasia within the follicle, creating adherent hyperkeratotic plugs that are resistant to expression.

PUVA therapy can cause acne also known as "acne aestivalis" as it often followed a Mediterranean holiday in sun, "Majorca acne".

Tropical Acne

Tropical acne is a follicular acneiform eruption that results from exposure to extreme heat. Usually it occurs in tropical climates or secondary to scorching occupational environments, as in furnace workers.

Historically, tropical acne caused significant morbidity among military troops. Markedly inflamed nodulocystic acne involving the trunk and buttocks is typically seen, and secondary staphylococcal infection is a frequent complication.

Treatment is often of limited efficacy until the patient returns to a more moderate climate.

Pseudoacne of the Transverse Nasal Crease

The transverse nasal crease is a horizontal anatomical demarcation line found in the lower third of the nose which corresponds to the separation point between the alar cartilage and the triangular cartilage. Milia, cysts and comedones can line up along this fold. These acne-like lesions arise during early childhood prior to the onset of puberty.

Treatment consists of surgical expression.

Idiopathic Facial Aseptic Granuloma

This chronic, painless, solitary nodule with an acneiform appearance can develop on the cheeks of young children.

Histopathologic evaluation reveals a dermal lymphohistiocytic infiltrate with foreign body-type giant cells.

Cultures are typically negative (70% of patients) and the lesions do not respond to antibiotic therapy.

They eventually resolve spontaneously after an average of 11 months, without treatment.[9]

Childhood Flexural Comedones

This recently described entity is characterized by discrete, double orifice comedones localized to the axillae and, less commonly, the groin. The majority of patients have a single lesion and the average age at diagnosis is 6 years, with boys and girls equally affected.[10]

There is no association with other signs of hidradenitis suppurativa, acne vulgaris or precocious puberty. In most cases, the flexural comedones are discovered incidentally in patients presenting with other dermatologic conditions.

Pityrosporum Folliculitis

It is caused by a host reaction to the yeast *Malassezia furfur*, previously named *Pityrosporum ovale*, a normal human skin commensal organism. It appears primarily on the trunk and upper extremities of adolescents and young adults. Unlike acne vulgaris, it is pruritic, without comedones.

Diagnosis is typically made clinically, although the yeast and hyphae can be observed in biopsy specimens in the widened follicular ostia along with keratinous material, and occasionally, rupture of the follicular wall may occur.

Patients may be treated with topical leave-on, wash-off, or systemic antifungal therapy.

Eosinophilic Pustular Folliculitis (EPF)

It is a disease of unclear etiology, thought to be an allergic hypersensitivity. It appears as a recurrent pruritic papulopustular eruption on the face, trunk, and extremities. Histopathology reveals a predominantly perifollicular infiltration of eosinophils with some mononuclear cells and subcorneal pustules composed of eosinophils.

Three main types exist:

1. Infantile form
2. HIV associated which is most common on extrafacial sites, and
3. Classic Ofuji disease in immunocompetent patients that occurs specially in Japan predominantly involving face. Patients may also demonstrate blood eosinophilia and leukocytosis.

Pathophysiology: The cause is not clearly understood but hypothesis suggests that it occurs as hypersensitivity reaction to *Malassezia* spp., *Demodex* spp. or sebaceous gland derived lipids. The fluid from pustules is sterile and rich in chemotactic factors.

Histology suggests perifollicular and perivascular eosinophilic infiltration. Mild to moderate eosinophilia is also seen with HIV-induced EPF.

Treatment modalities and results vary greatly. Options include potent topical corticosteroids and topical tacrolimus or pimecrolimus, indomethacin, nb-UVB phototherapy as first line management while oral corticosteroids and antimicrobials, dapsone, isotretinoin, and cetirizine as second line drugs. Indomethacin is the treatment of choice for classic Ofuji disease.

REFERENCES

1. Bahbouhi I, Aboudourib M, Hocar O, Amal S. Vitamin B12 induced acneiform eruption. Heliyon. 2023 May 20;9(5):e16120. doi: 10.1016/j.heliyon.2023.e16120. PMID: 37305488; PMCID: PMC10256894.
2. Rothstein G, Clarkson DR, Larsen W, et al. Effect of lithium on neutrophil mass and production. N Engl J Med 1978; 298:173–80.
3. Madke B, Gole P, Kumar P, Khopkar U. Dermatological side effects of epidermal growth factor receptor inhibitors: 'PRIDE' Complex. Indian J Dermatol. 2014 May;59(3):271-4. doi: 10.4103/0019-5154.131398. PMID: 24891659; PMCID: PMC4037949.
4. DeWitt CA, Siroy AE, Stone SP. Acneiform eruptions associated with epidermal growth factor receptor–targeted chemotherapy. J of the American Academy of Dermatology 2007 March;56(3)500–5.
5. Hengge UR, Ruzicka T, Schwartz RA, Cork MJ. Adverse effects of topical glucocorticosteroids. J Am Acad Dermatol 2006 Jan; 54(1):1–15.
6. Lynch TJ, Jr, Kim ES, Eaby B, et al. Epidermal growth factor receptor inhibitor-associated cutaneous toxicities: an evolving paradigm in clinical management. Oncologist. 2007;12:610–21. [PubMed]
7. McDonagh AJ, Gawkrodger DJ, Walker AE. Chloracne-study of an outbreak with new clinical observations. Clin Exp Dermatol. 1993;18:523–5.
8. Heydenreich G, Larsen PO. Iododerma after high dose urography in an oliguric patient. Br J Dermatol 1977; 97:567–9.
9. Boralevi F, Leaute-Labreze C, Lepreux S, et al. Idiopathic facial aseptic granuloma: a multicentre prospective study of 30 cases. Br J Dermatol. 2007;156:705–8.
10. Larralde M, Abad M, Muñoz AS, et al. Childhood flexural comedones: a new entity. Arch Dermatol. 2007;143:909–11. https://www.ncbi.nlm.nih.gov/pmc/articles/PMC4037949/
11. Biswal, Anisha & Samal, Abhipsa & Panda, Maitreyee. (2023). Tofacitinib-induced acne in a patient of vitiligo vulgaris: A case report. Cosmoderma. 10.25259/CSDM_81_2023.

CHAPTER

9

Differential Diagnosis

The age of onset, morphology and distribution make the diagnosis of acne quite straightforward, however, there are number of skin conditions which should be kept in mind.

NEONATAL AND INFANCY

During the neonatal period, acne must be differentiated from other common dermatoses.

Sebaceous Hyperplasia

This commonly presents as transient yellowish papules on the cheeks, nose and forehead. It occurs in majority of the healthy neonates.

Miliaria Rubra/Crystallina

It is the temporary obstruction of the eccrine ducts leading to formation of small inflammatory papules and occasionally pustules.

Milia

Small, white papules often appear on the cheeks and nose of neonates, generally resolve within a few months.

Sterile Transient Neonatal Pustulosis

It is benign condition. Present with sterile pustules without erythema over forehead, neck, lower back and shins. It resolves by its own.

Erythema toxicum neonatorum

Onset of ETN is usually at 24–48 hours of birth. Presents as erythematous papules, pustules, macules. Mostly seen in term infants.

Scabies

It present with papules, nodules, pustules, crusted lesions, vesicles and burrows over face, palms, soles, axillae and groin.

Congenital Candidiasis

It is usually present with widespread erythema, papulopustular lesions. Often associated with *in utero* infections, foreign body in cervix/uterus. More common in premature infants.

ADOLESCENTS AND YOUNG

Nevus Comedonicus

It is type of epidermal nevus. Usually develop before 10 years of age. It presents as a grouped, dilated follicular openings with dark keratin plugs. If it is present on face then it can be confused with grade 1 acne (open comedones).

Gram-negative Folliculitis

It is caused by Gram-negative organisms such as Klebsiella, *Escherichia coli, Serratia marcescens, Proteus mirabilis* or *Pseudomonas aeruginosa*. It can occur as a complication of long-term oral or topical antibiotic therapy used to treat acne. It has also been reported in HIV-positive patients.

Clinical features include a sudden eruption of multiple small follicular pustules or occasionally nodular lesions, most frequently localized around the perioral or perinasal skin.

Malassezia Folliculitis

Malassezia folliculitis is due to proliferation of the yeast within the hair follicles presenting frequently on the upper trunk as a monomorphic acne like eruption, viz. papules or pustules which may itch.

Scalp Folliculitis

Scalp folliculitis is an inflammatory disorder of the hair follicles characterized by small itchy pustules on the scalp often around the hairline. It results from an inflammatory reaction to microorganisms including bacteria (*P. acnes, Staphylococcus aureus*), yeasts (*Malassezia* spp.) and mites (*Demodex folliculorum*).

Perioral Dermatitis

It usually presents as papules and pustules on an erythematous and/or scaling base localized symmetrically around the mouth with a clear zone around the vermillion border. Lesions frequently itch in perioral dermatitis and no comedones are evident.

Milia

Milia are intraepidermal keratin cysts predominantly infraorbital in distribution. Closed comedones, i.e. whiteheads may be confused with milia (Fig. 9.1).

Syringomas

Syringomas are non-inflammatory papules that occur primarily around the eyelids and upper cheeks (Fig. 9.2). Histology demonstrates a dense fibrous stroma with dilated cystic spaces.

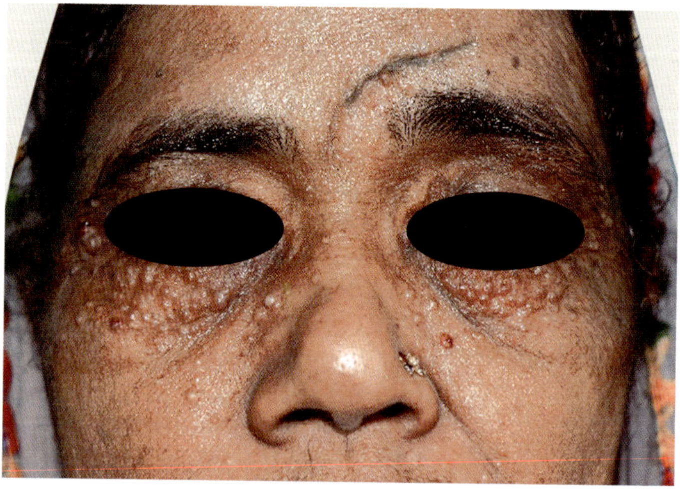

Fig. 9.1: Milia

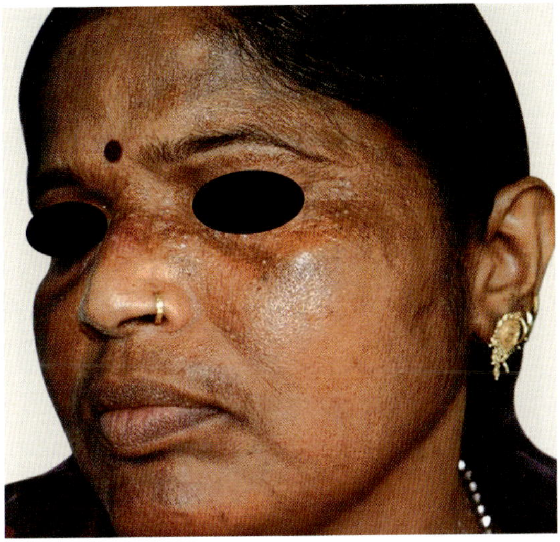

Fig. 9.2: Syringoma

Fibrofolliculomas

Fibrofolliculomas are 2–4 mm dome-shaped papules seen most commonly on the face, neck and upper trunk. They are characteristically seen in Birt-Hogg-Dube (BHD) syndrome.

Adenoma Sebaceum

Adenoma sebaceum are small translucent vascular papules symmetrically distributed over the central face. Multiple lesions are associated with tuberous sclerosis (Fig. 9.3).

Trichoepithelioma

Trichoepithelioma is a rare benign skin lesion that originates from hair follicles. Trichoepitheliomas are mostly seen in the scalp, nose, forehead, and upper lip. These skin lesions originate from benign proliferation of epithelial-mesenchymal origin cells. Trichoepitheliomas may be divided into the multiple familial trichoepithelioma, solitary trichoepithelioma and desmoplastic trichoepithelioma. It usually appears as multiple lesions in the autosomal dominant type or as an individual flesh colored papule or nodule measuring 2 to 8 mm in the sporadic type (Fig. 9.4).

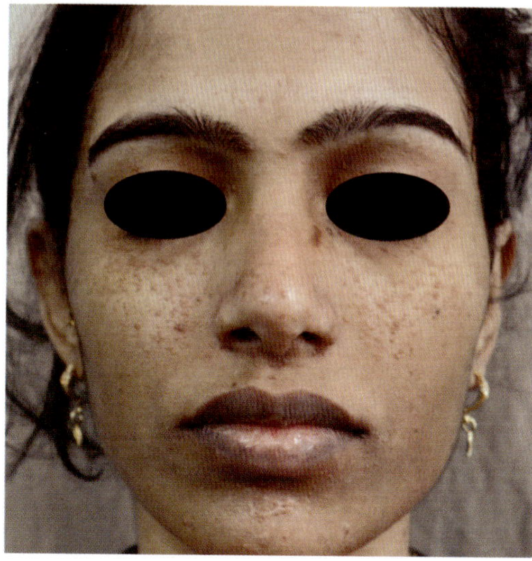

Fig. 9.3: Adenoma sebaceum

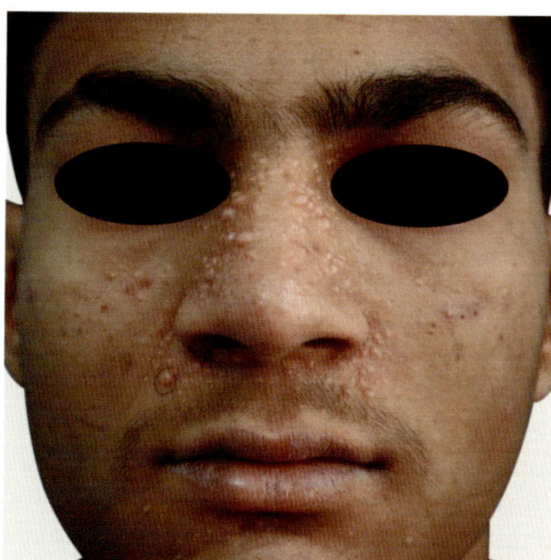

Fig. 9.4: Familial trichoepithelioma

Hidradenitis Suppurativa

Hidradenitis suppurativa is a chronic disease that affects the axillae, breasts, genital and perianal areas. There are open

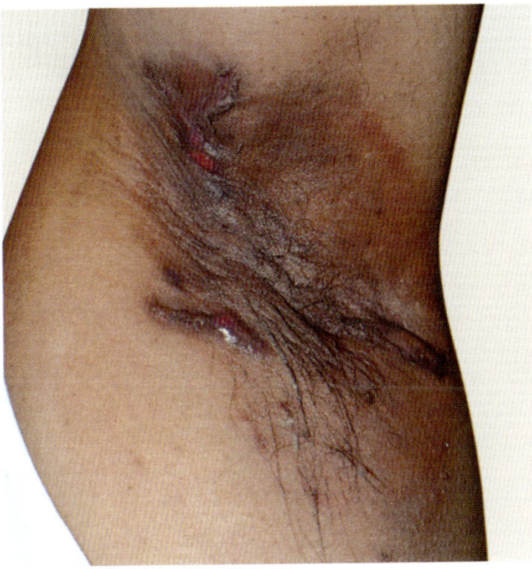

Fig. 9.5: Hidradenitis suppurativa

comedones (often polyporous), deep nodules, large abscesses, sinus tracts and scarring (Fig. 9.5). It is primarily a disorder of follicular occlusion. Family history is generally present and the onset is usually in late adolescence and the disease prevalence gradually decreases with increasing age.

Sebaceous (Epidermoid) Cysts and Steatocystoma Multiplex

Sebaceous cysts are multiple smooth yellow dermal swellings varying from a few millimetres to 20 mm in size distributed on the arms, chest, neck and axillae and appear and/or enlarge at puberty. Multiple true sebaceous cysts occur as so called steatocystoma multiplex (SM), a naevoid condition that histologically shows a mixture of a keratinizing epithelium and sebaceous lobules attached to the epidermis by a thin epidermal strand.

Dowling-Degos Disease (DDD)

Dowling-Degos Disease is autosomal dominant disorder. It is associated with genetic mutations in genes like KRT5 and POFUT1. Onset occurs in late adolescence or early adulthood. One of the distinguishing features of Dowling-Degos disease is the

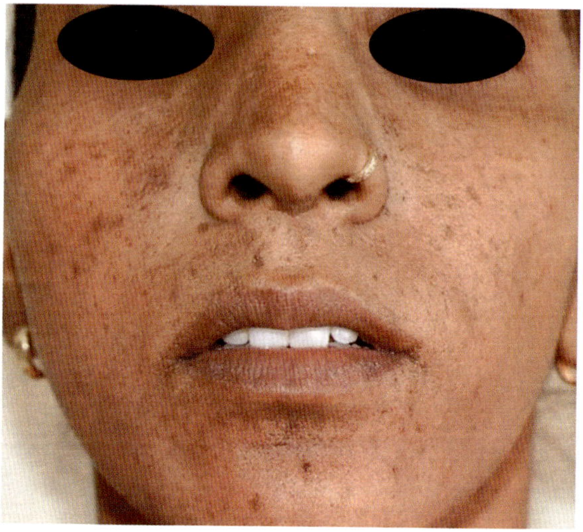

Fig. 9.6: Pitted perioral scars and lentigo like macules over face in Dowling-Degos disease

formation of a reticulated (net-like) pattern of lesions on the skin. The lesions are commonly found in flexural areas, including the neck, groin, armpits, and skin folds. However, they may also occur on the face, back, and other parts of the body. Lentigo like brown papules and macules, comedone-like lesions on back and neck, pitted perioral scars and palmar pits are present. DDD is linked to other skin conditions like hidradenitis suppurativa and pilonidal cysts (Fig 9.6).

MIDDLE AGE

Rosacea

Rosacea may occasionally be mistaken for inflammatory acne. Rosacea usually occurs in an older age group of patients, i.e. 30–50 years of age, and lacks comedones or scarring and rarely affects the trunk. Papules and pustules, telangiectasias are prominent on the face and chin (Fig. 9.7). The presence of facial flushing and specific triggers, including heat, spicy food or alcohol, are more commonly associated with rosacea. Rosacea patients may also have ocular involvement.

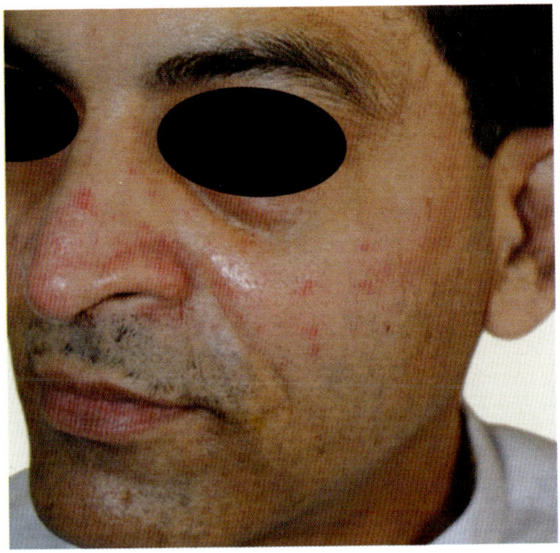

Fig. 9.7: Rosacea

Ectopic Sebaceous Glands

Fordyce spots are heterotopic sebaceous glands that are multiple, and appear as symmetrical discrete yellow papules occurring around the vermilion border of the lips or within the oral mucosa. These are present in 25% of the population over the age of 35 years and are usually asymptomatic but can be disfiguring.

Folliculitis Keloidalis

It is an unusual chronic form of folliculitis affecting the nape of the neck and associated with cicatricial alopecia, more common in black males. The lesions present as small itchy raised papules within or close to hair bearing areas of the occiput, secondary infection with *Staphylococcus aureus* can ensue. The chronic process results in hairless scarring. Tufted hairs may be present representing multiple hair shafts emerging from single follicular openings.

Lupus miliaris disseminatus faciei (LMDF)

LMDF is primarily an idiopathic granulomatous disease affecting facial skin, particularly the eyelids. LMDF can be seen across a wide range of ages, with the most common occurrence

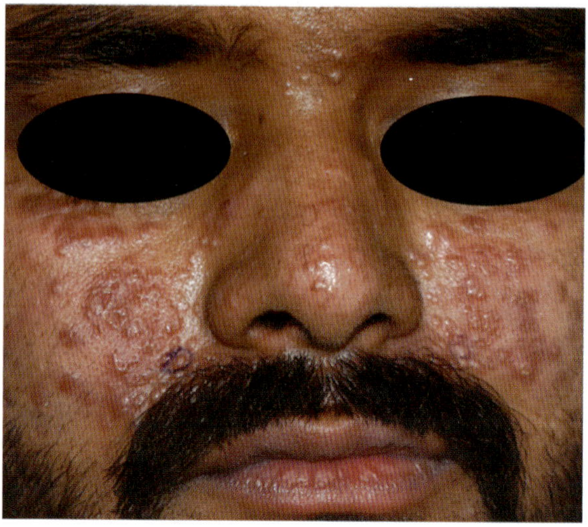

Fig. 9.8: Lupus miliaris disseminated faciei

in young adults (the average age in one series was 33 years) and is rare in older adults. A clear gender predilection has not been established. Patients often present with a relatively abrupt onset of asymptomatic discrete red, yellow, brown, or skin-colored papules or nodules, which are occasionally pustular and symmetrically distributed predominantly on facial skin (Fig. 9.8); these often predominate in the central face and are follicular or nonfollicular. The lower eyelids are most characteristically involved and the forehead, cheeks, nose, upper lips, ears, chin, or neck involvement is common. Co-morbidities have not generally been reported in association with LMDF.[3]

ELDERLY

Favre-Racouchot Syndrome

Multiple open and closed comedones occurring on periorbital and malar areas in elderly people in the context of chronic sun exposure. UVR results in solar damage to the supporting dermis causing the pilosebaceous duct to become distended with impacted corneocytes. Histology demonstrates increased elastic tissue with thickened and tortuous fibres in the upper and mid-dermis (Fig. 9.9).

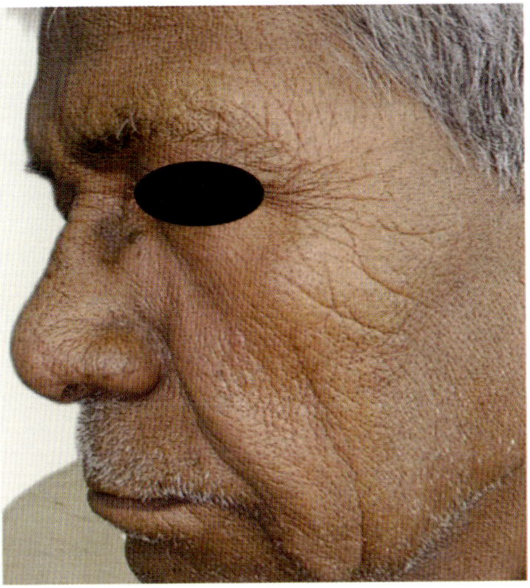

Fig. 9.9: Favre-Racouchot syndrome

Sebaceous Gland Hyperplasia

Sebaceous gland hyperplasia is a benign proliferation of the sebaceous and producing yellow/pink lesions 1–3 mm in diameter on the face.

Sebaceous Adenoma

This is a benign tumor composed of incompletely differentiated sebaceous cells. It occurs in both sexes, predominantly in the elderly on the face or scalp. The waxy pink/yellow tumors are usually 10 mm or less in size and may form ulcerative plaques.

Sebaceous Carcinoma

This is a rare malignant tumor arising from the sebaceous glands, common in men over the age of 40 years. It presents as a firm solitary yellow-orange lesion usually on the face and scalp.

Differential Diagnosis of Acne at a Glance

- Comedones
- Contact acne
- Acne exacerbated by systemic steroids or anabolic steroids

- Trichostasis spinulosa
- Favre-Racouchot disease
- Nevus comedonicus
- Basaloid follicular hamartoma syndrome
- Familial dyskeratotic comedones
- Radiation-induced comedones
- Dilated pore of Winer
- Follicular spines
- Closed comedonal
- Milia
- Osteoma cutis
- Sebaceous hyperplasia
- Syringomas
- Trichoepitheliomas
- Trichodiscomas, fibrofolliculoma
- Eruptive vallus hair cysts, steatocystoma multiplex
- Colloid milia
- Contact acne
- Follicular mucinosis
- Inflammatory
- Rosacea
- Perioral dermatitis
- Folliculitis-culture negative normal flora, staphylococcal, Gram-negative, eosinophilic, pityrosporum.
- Acne or acneform eruptions due to topical or systemic corticosteroids, anabolic steroids or other medications (e.g. lithium).
- Pseudofolliculitis barbae
- Furuncle/carbuncle
- Neutrophilic dermatosis and neutrophilic eccrine hidradenitis
- Neonatal acne
- Miliaria rubra
- Solid facial edema secondary to acne vulgaris
- Solid facial edema secondary to rosacea
- Melkersson-Rosenthal syndrome
- Sarcoidosis

- Lepromatous leprosy
- Lymphomas
- Scleromyxedema
- Autoimmune connective tissue disease (e.g. dermatomyositis, lupus erythematosus, Still's diseases).

REFERENCES

1. Alison M. Layton, E. Anne Eady, Christos C. Zouboulis. Department of Dermatology, Harrogate and District NHS Foundation Trust, Harrogate, UK, Departments of Dermatology, Venereology, Allergology and Immunology, Dessau Medical Center, Dessau, Germany, Acne, Rook's Textbook of Dermatology, ninth edition.
2. Andrea L Zaenglein, Diane M Thiboutot. Acne vulgaris, Jean Bolognia, Textbook of Dermatology, Third Edition.
3. Slater N, Rapini RP. Lupus miliaris disseminatus faciei 2024.

CHAPTER
10

Systemic Therapy

Oral therapy is generally started when there is a significant inflammatory component and/or the acne is extensive and/or topical applications alone are ineffective.

Oral medications are:

1. Antibiotics
2. Retinoids
3. Hormonal therapy
4. Zinc
5. Newer oral therapies

ORAL ANTIBIOTICS

Oral antibiotics are the most widely prescribed agents in acne and are indicated for moderate to severe inflammatory acne, and/or extensive truncal acne.

Different oral antibiotics used in acne are:

1. Cyclines
2. Macrolides
3. Trimethoprim
4. Cephalosporins

Cyclines

Are considered to be drug of choice.

Mechanism of Action

a. **Antimicrobial:** They are mainly bacteriostatic and they do so by inhibiting bacterial protein synthesis by binding to the 30S ribosomal subunit of *P. acnes*. At higher concentration, bactericidal.

b. **Anti-inflammatory:** This action is seen at a dose lower than required for antimicrobial activity (sub-antimicrobial dose). Acts by inhibiting production of free fatty acids from *P. acnes*, decreasing matrix metalloproteinase activity, inhibiting leukocyte chemotaxis and reducing production of proinflammatory cytokines (e.g. TNF-α, IL-1), scavenger effect against reactive oxygen species (ROS).

Doxycycline can inhibit MMP-2, MMP-3, MMP-8, MMP-9, and MMP-13, which expression is increased in acne.

It also involved inhibition of trypsin-like serine protease in the skin through the inhibition of kallikrein-5, which is also involved in skin inflammation. Also decreases levels of TNF-α, IL-1β, IL-6, and IL-8 by suppressing activation of the NF-kB pathway and of TNF-α converting enzyme (TACE).

Different drugs belonging to this group are:

- **1st generation:** Tetracycline.
- **2nd generation:** Doxycycline, Minocycline, Lymecycline.
- **3rd generation:** Sarecycline.

Dosing

Tetracycline (initial dose—500 mg QID, maintenance dose—250–500 mg per day) should be taken 1 hour before or 2 hours after meals/empty stomach (since absorption is reduced by 50% when taken with food).

Doxycycline (antimicrobial dose—100 mg, subantimicrobial dose—40 mg/day) and minocycline (100 mg) can be taken with (to reduce symptoms GI upset) food.

Lymecycline and doxycycline should be used in preference to minocycline.[1]

Sarecycline has been approved by the FDA for treatment of moderate to severe acne vulgaris in 2018 in patients above 9 years of age. Due to higher selectivity for *C. acnes* compared to older-generation tetracyclines, there is a lower risk of developing bacterial resistance during treatment. It showed good effectiveness in the treatment of severe facial and truncal acne, with a relatively low rate of side effects and good tolerability.[1]

Weight based dosage of sarecycline:[2]

- **33–54 kg:** 60 mg OD
- **55–84 kg:** 100 mg OD
- **85–136 mg:** 150 mg OD

Contraindications

1. Pregnancy
2. Children under 12 years of age (risk of teeth discoloration)
3. Renal impairment (except doxycycline, which is excreted via hepatobiliary tract).

Common Side Effects

1. Nausea, vomiting, abdominal pain
2. Phototoxicity (doxycycline)
3. Photo-onycholysis (minocycline) and pseudoporphyria
4. Hyperpigmentation—diffuse and muddy-brown accentuated in sun-exposed areas, bluish discoloration of scars (including those due to acne) and normal skin (in particular on the shins), grayish blue discoloration of the oral mucosa, sclera, nails and teeth (more with minocycline).
5. Deposition in the teeth and bones in children, causing discoloration and hypoplasia of the teeth and stunted growth.[3]

Serious Side Effects

1. Serum sickness-like reactions
2. Esophageal ulcerations
3. Pseudomembranous enterocolitis
4. Blood dyscrasias
5. Pseudotumor cerebri—risk of which may be increased when given together with a systemic retinoid
6. Nephrotoxicity

Drug Interactions

Effects of other drugs on tetracyclines:

1. Antacids, H2 blockers, proton pump inhibitors decrease absorption.
2. Anticonvulsants reduce t1/2 of tetracyclines.

Effects of tetracyclines on other drugs:

1. Raise serum levels of digoxin, lithium and warfarin
2. Decrease requirement of insulin

Macrolides

Due to the emergence of antibiotic-resistant strains of *P. acnes*, macrolides nowadays are not preferred.

Limited indications where macrolides are used are:

1. In pregnancy, oral erythromycin is thought to be safe although there is no data available evaluating chronic use over prolonged periods in pregnancy.[4] It should be taken on empty stomach.
2. Children (8–12 years).

Mechanism of Action

1. Antimicrobial—by inhibiting bacterial protein synthesis after binding to the 50S ribosomal subunit, these act as bacteriostatic drugs.
2. Anti-inflammatory

Azithromycin—intermittent dosing schedules can also be used.

It is not advisable to use as widespread resistance is reported to it.

Common Side Effects

1. Gastrointestinal intolerance (more with erythromycin)
2. Intrahepatic cholestasis in adults, risk increases during pregnancy (especially with erythromycin estolate)

Rare and Serious Side Effects

1. Acute generalized exanthematous pustulosis
2. Stevens-Johnson syndrome
3. Toxic epidermal necrolysis
4. Vasculitis

Contraindications

1. Hypersensitivity to the drug
2. Hepatic dysfunction

Drug Interactions

Due to CYP3A4 inhibition, increased risk of

1. Torsades de pointes
2. Toxicity of multiple drugs by increasing serum levels, e.g. anticonvulsants, oral contraceptive pills, cyclosporine, etc. Azithromycin has improved gastrointestinal tolerance and a little potential for significant metabolism-based drug interactions.[5]

Clindamycin

It is highly lipophilic drug and very effective in acne but adverse effects, including diarrhea (5–20%), and potential pseudomembranous colitis from overgrowth of *Clostridium difficile* has discouraged its use.

Co-trimoxazole

It is a synergistic combination of sulfamethoxazole and trimethoprim.

It is indicated in acne resistant to cyclines and macrolides.

Mechanism of Action

It acts by inhibiting 2 steps in folic acid synthesis within bacteria. Sulfamethoxazole inhibits dihydropteroate synthetase and conversion of PABA to folic acid, while trimethoprim blocks dihydrofolate reductase and thus conversion of dihydrofolate to tetrahydrofolate.

Dosing

6–12 mg/kg of trimethoprim and 30–60 mg/kg of sulfamethoxazole 12 hourly. Ideally co-trimoxazole contains 80 mg of trimethoprim and 400 mg of sulfamethoxazole. Double strength dose contains 160 mg and 800 mg of above drugs respectively.

Side Effects

Majority due to sulphonamides

1. Adverse cutaneous drug eruptions—ranging from morbilliform eruptions, urticaria, FDE to Stevens-Johnson syndrome, toxic epidermal necrolysis.

2. GI upset, glossitis and stomatitis, dizziness and headaches.
3. Megaloblastic anemia

Contraindications

1. Hypersensitivity
2. Third trimester of pregnancy and in lactating patients (risk of kernicterus in newborn).
3. Porphyria
4. G6PD deficiency (risk of hemolytic anemia).

Drug Interactions

1. Increase serum levels oral hypoglycemics and warfarin.
2. Decrease protein binding and renal clearance of methotrexate, thus increasing risk of mtx toxicity.

Emerging Antibiotic Resistance

Recently, multiple published literature is showing *P. acne* antibacterial resistance, especially with macrolide group, due to point mutation in 23 sRNA.

Cross-resistance seen amongst erythromycin and clindamycin. *P. acne* resistance is easily disseminated and can be detected in around 50% of close contacts of acne patients. Therefore, antibiotic monotherapy is never to be indicated.

Emergence of resistance in different drugs is as follows:

- Erythromycin > Doxycycline, tetracycline
- Cotrimoxazole > Minocycline.[6]

When to suspect antibacterial resistant *P. acnes*

1. Failure to respond to antibiotic therapy.
2. Worsening of acne despite regular antibiotic therapy.
3. Prolonged monotherapy of topical and oral antibiotic therapy.

Strategy to avoid Propionibacterium resistance

1. Avoid inappropriate use of topical and systemic antibiotics.
2. If extending the duration of oral antibiotics, utilize combination therapy.
3. If repeated courses of antibiotics are required and the initial clinical response is favorable, reuse the same drug.

4. Avoid prescribing different oral and topical antibiotics concomitantly.
5. Consider using topical retinoids and non-antibiotic antimicrobials wherever possible.
6. Topical benzoyl peroxide (BPO) can be used for 7 days between antibiotic courses.
7. Check medical adherence.

ORAL RETINOIDS

Retinoids are synthetic derivatives of vitamin A.

Classification

1. **1st generation:** Ttretinoin, isotretinoin, alitretinoin, micronized isotretinoin.
2. **2nd generation:** Acitretin, etretinate.
3. **3rd generation:** Bexarotene, adapalene, tazarotene.
4. **4th generation:** Trifarotene.

Isotretinoin (13-cis-retinoic acid) is FDA approved for nodulocystic and recalcitrant acne (i.e. not responding to other conventional treatment options or with tendency for scarring).

Other Indications

1. Gram-negative folliculitis
2. Acne fulminans
3. Relapsing acne
4. Acne with severe psychological distress

Mechanism of Action

- Oral isotretinoin causes shrinkage of sebaceous glands and a marked attenuation of sebum secretion. The decrease in sebum results in the inhibition of the sebum-dependent bacterium Propionibacterium acne, which is a key promoter of inflammation in acne vulgaris.
- Oral isotretinoin also inhibits comedogenesis by fostering keratinocyte differentiation and by normalizing desquamation.
- Isotretinoin is the only treatment that has been shown to induce long-term remissions in acne as it affects almost all stages of pathogenesis.

Dosing

Isotretinoin has to be taken with meal (fatty), since it increases bioavailability.

In 1989, concept of cumulative dosing was introduced by Harms et al. It refers to the total amount of oral isotretinoin taken by the patient over the entire course, divided by the body weight (mg/kg body weight). Several studies have indicated that post-therapy relapse is minimized by a treatment course amounting to a total of at least 120 mg/kg, with no further therapeutic gain beyond about 150 mg/kg.[7]

Dose: 0.5 to 2 mg/kg/day for 3–5 months period.

It takes 1–3 months to show complete therapeutic effect.

Low relapse rates are observed after stopping the drug. Multiple courses can be given to a patient who was started on low dose (0.5 mg/kg/day).

Side Effects

1. Teratogenicity
2. Mucocutaneous-cheilitis, xeroderma, dry eyes and nose.
3. Arthralgia
4. Hypertriglyceridemia, raised liver function enzymes.
5. DISH (diffuse interstitial skeletal hyperostosis) syndrome.
6. Depression, suicidal tendencies.
7. Pseudotumor cerebri, if given along with tetracyclines.

Contraindications

1. Pregnancy and lactation
2. Hypersensitivity

Caution

Males on isotretinoin therapy: Blood transfusion to be avoided till 1 month after stopping treatment.

i-PLEDGE programme: Drug Safety Program was launched in 2006.

Four companies that manufacture isotretinoin and the FDA agreed to establish a federal registry in which it is mandatory that all patients receiving isotretinoin are enrolled.

Wholesalers, pharmacies, prescribers, and patients are part of this registry, and a certain set of requirements must be met before an isotretinoin prescription can be filled. The program dictates that women of childbearing potential should use two forms of contraception while on isotretinoin. For men or women not of childbearing potential, the system must still be accessed at the time of each prescription to confirm counselling.

Drug Interactions

1. Antitubercular drugs and anticonvulsants reduce the blood levels of isotretinoin.
2. Macrolides increase blood levels of isotretinoin due to CYP 3A4 inhibition.

Monitoring Guidelines: Baseline and Follow-up

1. Serum pregnancy test (in women of childbearing potential) (repeated monthly).
2. Complete blood count (CBC)
3. Liver function tests (if baseline is normal, no need to repeat).
4. Lipid profile (monitor monthly for the 1st 3–6 months, then every 3 months).

ROLE OF MICRONIZED ISOTRETINOIN IN MICRO MANAGEMENT OF ACNE

Acne is a challenging dermatological disorder that often needs systemic therapy. Isotretinoin, a derivative of vitamin A, due to its profound effectiveness has been the gold standard treatment for decades. Over the years, different dosing strategies and formulations have emerged to optimize efficacy while minimizing side effects.

However, traditional isotretinoin formulations require administration with a high-fat meal to optimize absorption and can be associated with significant adverse effects. The advent of micronized isotretinoin offers a promising advancement, providing improved bioavailability, reduced food dependence, along with a comparative improvement in its safety profile.

Isotretinoin (13-cis-retinoic acid) is an oral retinoid that targets multiple acne pathophysiological mechanisms, including:

- Reduction in size of sebaceous gland and sebum production.
- Normalization of follicular keratinization and preventing formation of microcomedone
- Reduces inflammatory cytokines and immune responses contributing to acne.

Notwithstanding its effectiveness, conventional formulations of isotretinoin have limitations on account of variable absorption, dependence on food intake, and mucocutaneous and systemic side effects like alterations in lipid profile and liver function test.

Micronized isotretinoin is an optimized version of standard isotretinoin. It undergoes a specialized micronization process that increases the surface area of the drug particles, thereby enhancing dissolution and absorption. Compared to traditional formulations, micronized isotretinoin offers the following advantages

- Improved bioavailability-better drug absorption at lower doses.
- Reduced dependence on food intake-reater dosing flexibility.
- Potentially fewer adverse effects, particularly mucocutaneous and lipid-related side effects.
- Lower doses required for similar efficacy
- More stable drug levels → Consistent acne suppression

A pharmacokinetic study compared micronized isotretinoin (32 mg) and Low dose-isotretinoin (40 mg) in fed and fasted conditions. Key outcomes included

- In-fed conditions, micronized isotretinoin: bioequivalent to Low dose -isotretinoin.
- In fasting conditions: Micronized isotretinoin had twice the absorption of Low dose isotretinoin, suggesting superior fasting bioavailability.
- Minimal impact of food on absorption, making it more convenient for patients.

These findings underscore micronized isotretinoin's potential to eliminate the need for food-dependent dosing, which has been a major drawback of traditional isotretinoin formulations.

Six hundred patients participated in a randomized, double-blind, multicenter study comparing micronized isotretinoin (0.4 mg/kg once daily, in a fasting state) with standard isotretinoin (1.0 mg/kg in divided doses with food). The results demonstrated clinical equivalence between the two formulations in terms of reduction of acne lesion

Notably, patients on micronized isotretinoin exhibited fewer adverse events, including:

- Less occurrence of mucocutaneous effects, such as dry skin, nosebleeds, and eye irritation.
- Lower frequency of hypertriglyceridemia
- Similar psychiatric safety profile, with no significant increase in mood disturbances or depression.

The introduction of micronized isotretinoin,a next-generation formulation represents a significant step forward in acne management that overcomes many limitations of traditional isotretinoin therapy. Its enhanced bioavailability, better dosing flexibility and patient compliance, reduced food dependence, and improved safety profile make it an attractive option for treating acne. Ongoing studies will further refine its role in clinical practice, but early data strongly support its use as a more effective and convenient treatmen-t for patients with acne.

HORMONAL THERAPY

Systemic hormonal medications are indicated in female patients with acne in the following conditions:

1. When obvious cutaneous signs of hyperandrogenism are seen, e.g. SAHA syndrome.
2. Recalcitrant acne
3. PCOS

Different hormonal preparations

1. Oral contraceptives
2. Low-dose corticosteroids

Oral Contraceptives

Are fixed dose combinations of estrogen (especially ethinyl estradiol) and progesterone.

Mechanism of Action

Estrogens decrease sebum production by both locally at the level of the sebaceous gland, by suppressing excess androgen secretion by polycystic ovaries.

The two hormones, estrogen and androgen, normally balance each other in women. Androgens trigger sebum oil production. When estrogen levels are low and androgen levels are high, the androgens can overstimulate the sebaceous glands and cause too much oil production. In the second half of the menstrual cycle, androgen levels are naturally high and estrogen is naturally low, which is why many women get premenstrual acne. In other women, especially those with polycystic ovary syndrome (PCOS), hormone levels are far out of balance. These women are likely to have hormone-related acne all the time.

A significant portion of the circulating androgens is produced by the adrenal gland and the testes or ovaries. Besides sebaceous glands, other androgen-sensitive components of skin are hair follicles, sweat glands, epidermis, and dermis. These structures contain enzymes important in converting DHEA, DHEA-S, and androstenedione into the potent androgens dihydrotestosterone (DHT) and testosterone. DHT and testosterone are the major androgens that interact with the androgen receptors on sebaceous glands with DHT being 5 to 10 times more potent than testosterone. This conversion of inactive adrenal precursors to potent androgen occurs in sebaceous glands in the presence of several key steroidogenic enzymes: 3β-hydroxysteroid dehydrogenase (3β-HSD), 17β-hydro- xysteroid dehydrogenase (17β-HSD), and 5-reductase. 5-reductase is an important enzyme in androgen-dependent disorders, such as acne, male pattern baldness, and hirsutism.

Estrogen is known to suppress sebum production when given in sufficient amounts by giving a negative feedback to these enzymes. Other mechanisms for estrogen's effect include direct opposition effect on testosterone and inhibition of testosterone secretion.

Estrogen also provides negative feedback on the pituitary/ hypothalamus. That is, it inhibits the anterior pituitary's production of luteinizing hormone (LH) and follicle-stimulating hormone (FSH), thus decreasing ovarian production of the androgen, testosterone.

Estrogen administration increases sex hormone binding globulin, which binds serum testosterone, decreasing the amount of free testosterone available to bind with the androgen receptor. FDA approved combinations are:

1. Norgestimate + Ethinyl estradiol
2. Norethindrone acetate + Ethinyl estradiol

Dosing

To be given from first day of menstrual cycle till 21 days (3 week cycle).

Results are seen only after 3–4 cycles.

Side Effects

1. Nausea, weight gain
2. Breast tenderness, spotting
3. Thromboembolism

Low Dose Corticosteroids

Mechanism of action: Adrenal suppression thus reduces production of adrenal androgens.

Indication

Congenital adrenal hyperplasia (CAH). Late onset or non-classical CAH.

Dosing: Dexamethasone 0.25 mg HS for 6 months/0.5 mg HS for consecutive 3 months followed by 0.5 mg alternate nights for next 3 months. Prednisolone or deflazacort can also be used.

Anti-androgen and Androgen Receptor Blocker

Hormonal anti-androgen treatment is limited to female patients who present with additional signs of hyper-androgenism.

In addition, females with acne tarda, persistent acne recalcitrant to treatment, with concurrent wish of contraception, and as a requirement for a systemic isotretinoin treatment can be treated with hormonal antiandrogens.

Hormonal anti-androgen treatment is not a primary monotherapy for uncomplicated acne.

Mechanism of action: It inhibits peripheral action of androgen by blocking androgen receptor.

Different drugs with dosing:

1. **Cyproterone acetate:** 50–100 mg/day from the 5th to the 15th days of the menstrual cycle, for a 6-month period.
2. **Drospirenone:** 3 mg/day during the 21-day cycle along with 30 μg of ethinyl estradiol.
3. **Spironolactone:** 50–200 mg/day for 6 months.
4. **Flutamide:** 62.5–125 mg daily/ 250 mg BD.
5. **Finasteride:** 5 mg daily.

Spironolactone

Spironolactone is a synthetic steroidal androgen receptor blocker.

Mechanism of Action

1. Competition with testosterone and DHT for androgen receptors, thereby decreasing androgen-stimulated sebum production.
2. Inhibition of androgen synthesis decreasing type 2 17β-HSD, thereby halting the conversion of androstenedione to testosterone.
3. Inhibition of 5α-reductase, thus halting the conversion of testosterone to DHT
4. Increasing the level of SHBG

Dose: 50 to 200 mg daily.

Side effects: Hyperkalemia, headache, dizziness, drowsiness, and confusion, nausea, vomiting, anorexia, and diarrhea.

In men: Decreased libido, impotence, and gynecomastia.

In women: Menstrual irregularities and breast tenderness/ enlargement.

Cyproterone Acetate

Mechanism of action: It works by inhibiting the conversion of DHEA to androstenedione by blocking 3β-HSD activity. This leads to an overall decrease in testosterone with subsequent decrease in sebum production.

Dose: 50 to 100 mg/day.

Side effects: Breast tenderness, headache, nausea, and break-through bleeding.

Flutamide

Mechanism of action: It is converted to the potent metabolite 2-hydroxyflutamide, which selectively inhibits the binding of DHT to the androgen receptor.

Dose: 62.5 to 500 mg/day.

Side effects: Breast tenderness, gastrointestinal upset, hot flashes, and decreased libido. Hepatotoxicity is the most dangerous.

Ectopeptidase Inhibitors

These inhibit proliferation and enhance differentiation of sebocytes, also act as anti-inflammatory by IL-1 receptor antagonism and T-cell inhibition.

Ectopeptidases are ubiquitously expressed and have pleiotropic functions. Ectoenzymes, beyond their proteolytic activity, influence fundamental biological processes such as growth, apoptosis, differentiation, adhesion, motility, invasion, cell-cell interaction, angiogenesis, and transformation. The pharmacological inhibition of dipeptidyl peptidase IV as well as aminopeptidase, membrane alanyl- aminopeptidase (mAAP), affects growth, cytokine production, and typical functions of human peripheral T cells both *in vitro* and *in vivo*.

Inhibitors of DP IV have potent immunosuppressive and anti-inflammatory effects, hence potential in diseases hallmarked by hyperproliferation and inflammation such as acne, e.g. thiazolidine, actinonin, bestatin.[8]

IGF-1 Reducing Drugs

IGF-1 might be involved in acne induction or aggravation through upregulation of inflammatory biomarkers in sebaceous glands. Increased gene expression of NF-κB was observed in cultured sebocytes treated with IGF-1 upregulation of inflammatory biomarkers by IGF-1 might be mediated via the NF-κB signaling pathway.

IGF1 reducing drugs like Metformin can be considered for the treatment of acne.[9]

Metformin

Mechanism of action in acne: In the human body IGF-1 is strongly expressed on sebocytes and suprabasal cells of the sebaceous ducts with IGF-R being voraciously expressed in all regions of sebaceous glands. As a result of this expression, there is stimulation of lipogenesis in sebaceous glands which potentiates the occurrence of acne. Metformin reduces the level of IGF-1.

Indication: PCOS, HAIR-AN

Metformin works to balance the hormones and control the acne outbreaks.

Dose: 500 to 1000 mg twice daily.

Vitamin D

Vitamin D deficiency is more common among acne patients than those with clear skin.

Vitamin D may impact sebocytes by producing cathelicidin and defensins. These proteins have antibacterial properties.

P. acnes is a potent inducer of Th17, and vitamin D inhibits *P. acnes*-induced Th17 differentiation and inflammation.[23] Vitamin D may inhibit mTOR. mTOR is a protein that regulates cell growth and causes the skin to produce more oil and leads to blocked pores. Vitamin D does the opposite; it reduces mTOR activity in the skin.

Vitamin D may reduce the growth of the cells that produce sebum, which would reduce the amount of oil the skin produces.

Essential Fatty Acids

Acne patients have also been shown to have low levels of linoleic acid in their skin surface lipids. A corollary hypothesis holds that low concentrations of linolenate in sebum impose a state of essential fatty acid deficiency on the cells of the follicular epithelium and induce the characteristic response of hyperkeratosis.

EFA are powerful anti-inflammatory agents that control the amount of androgens in the body, thus reducing the amount of sebum and acne breakouts in the process.

Linoleic acid is an EFA that the sebaceous glands use as a normal component of sebum. It helps promote healthy skin. However, due to hereditary factors, high consumption of trans-fatty acids or low consumption of essential fatty acids, some people have a systemic deficiency of EFA and linoleic acid. This may be the main driving factor in causing acne and a few skin conditions.

Studies have shown that trans-fatty acid break down the body's supply of important and beneficial EFA. As a result, linoleic acid becomes unobtainable in the skin resulting into EFA deficiency. The sebaceous glands use oleic acid to produce sebum. This makes it desiccant, firmer, irritating and aggravating to the skin. It encourages clogging that causes blackheads, whiteheads and acne.

Zinc

Zinc reduces inflammatory response to bacteria. Zinc reduces keratinocyte activation. Zinc is a DHT blocker, hence, it reduces the effects of androgens on the skin. Zinc is a powerful antioxidant.

Topical zinc alone as well as in combination with other agents is effective due to its anti-inflammatory activity and ability to reduce *P. acnes* counts by inhibition of *P. acnes* lipases and free fatty acid levels.[10]

Best type of zinc supplement for acne is zinc picolinate.

Dose: 10–15 mg of zinc per day.

Zileuton[11]

Mechanism of action: Leukotriene B4 (LTB4) is considered to be a major player in the development of tissue inflammation in acne vulgaris. Synthesis of LTB4 is controlled by the enzyme 5-lipoxygenase. Zileuton blocks the activity of 5-lipoxygenase enzyme.

Inhibition of lipid synthesis, especially of pro- inflammatory lipids, is likely to be the major effect of Zileuton on sebaceous glands followed by reduction of inflammatory lesions in acne.

PPAR Receptor Inhibitors

Metformin and thiazolidinediones (rosiglitazone, pioglitazone) can decrease both fasting and stimulated plasma insulin levels and reduce insulin resistance through interaction with PPAR-γ.

Troglitazone, another member of the thiazolidinedione family, has been withdrawn from use because of liver toxicity.

Although pioglitazone and rosiglitazone have an improved safety profile in terms of liver toxicity, reports of increased cardiovascular morbidity should exclude these agents from anti-acne treatment.

In addition, they may induce hypoglycemia in normoglycemic subjects.

This leaves only metformin as an anti-acne drug with clinical potential for improvement of both hirsutism and acne in females with polycystic ovary syndrome.

Diet and Acne

The Paleolithic diet, reflecting our ancestral eating patterns, is proposed to influence acne by excluding processed foods, dairy, grains, and refined sugars and including vegetables, fruits, nuts and roots. This diet helps in acne by reducing inflammation.

Palmitic acid, abundant in sebaceous lipids, is crucial for the skin barrier but excess may contribute to inflammation. Oleic acid, with anti-inflammatory properties found in natural oils, may help regulate sebum production. Studies suggest formulations balancing palmitic and oleic acids could be beneficial. However, the complex relationship between diet and acne involves individual variations, with genetics and hormones playing pivotal roles.

Protein supplements including: Whey proteins, anabolic steroids and dietary supplements use for muscle building and weight loss can cause severe extensive new onset acne or flare of existing acne.[12]

REFERENCES

1. Tobiasz A, Nowicka D, Szepietowski JC. Acne vulgaris—Novel treatment options and factors affecting therapy adherence: A narrative review. Journal of Clinical Medicine. 2022 Dec 19;11(24):7535.
2. Grada A, Del Rosso JQ, Graber E, Bunick CG, Stein Gold L, Moore AY, Baldwin H, Obagi Z, Damiani G, Carrothers T, McNamee B. Sarecycline treatment for acne vulgaris: Rationale for weight-based dosing and limited impact of food intake on clinical efficacy. Dermatologic therapy. 2022 Mar;35(3):e15275.
3. Cohan S, Bevelander G, Tiamisc T. Growth-inhibition of prematures receiving tetracycline. Am J Dis Child. 1963; 105:1008.
4. Carraso DA, Vander Straten M, Tyring SK. A review of antibiotics in dermatology. J Cutan Med Surg 2002;6:128–50.
5. Raimer SS. New and emerging therapies in pediatric dermatology. Dermatol Clin.2000;18:73–8.
6. Hassanzadeh P, Bahamani M, Mehrabani D. Bacterial resistance to antibiotics in acne vulgaris: an in vitro study. Indian J Dermatol. 2008; 53:122–4.
7. Layton AM et al. Isotretinoin for acne vulgaris—10 years later: a safe and successful treatment. Br J Dermatol 1993;129(3):292–6.
8. Thieliez A, Reinhold D, Vetter R et al. Inhibitors of dipeptidyl peptidase IV and aminopeptidase N target major pathogenic steps in acne initiation. J Invest Dermatol.2007;127(5):1042–51.
9. Kim H, Moon SY, Sohn MY, Lee WJ. Insulin-like growth factor-1 increases the expression of inflammatory biomarkers and sebum production in cultured sebocytes. Ann Dermatol. 2017 Feb;29(1):20-25. doi: 10.5021/ad.2017.29.1.20. Epub 2017 Feb 3. PMID: 28223742; PMCID: PMC5318522
10. Gupta M, Mahajan VK, Mehta KS, Chauhan PS. Zinc therapy in dermatology: A Review. Dermatology Research and Practice. 2014;2014:709152. doi:10.1155/2014/709152.
11. Zouboulis CC. Zileuton, a new efficient and safe systemic anti- acne drug. Dermato-endocrinology. 2009;1(3):188–92.
12. Ambalal SM, Vyas HR. Cutaneous side effects of sports supplements. Indian Dermatology Online Journal. 2024 Mar 1;15(2):293–6.

CHAPTER

11

Topical Treatment

Topical treatment is the first line therapy in all grades of acne vulgaris and the treatment of choice for mild acne.

It has less potential side effects in comparison to oral treatment.

TOPICAL RETINOIDS

Topical retinoids target abnormal follicular epithelial hyperproliferation by reducing follicular plugging and formation of micro-comedones, thus resulting into overall reduction of non-inflammatory as well as inflammatory acne lesions. These also inhibit abnormal keratinocyte proliferation, improve differentiation and prevent the formation of precursor lesion.

TLR-2 when activated by *P. acnes* leads to upregulation of proinflammatory mediators **NF-κB**, IL-8, and IL-12. Topical retinoids inhibit this process and along with the prevention of pathogen-associated molecular pattern (PAMP), leading to further reduction of inflammation by inhibiting IL-1 release and reducing follicular wall permeability.[1]

By providing an aerobic environment, topical retinoids make the skin inhospitable for *P. acnes*. Adapalene, in addition, shows an anti-inflammatory effect by inhibiting the lipo-oxygenase pathway and chemotaxis and free oxygen radical release from neutrophils.

These are considered first-line treatment for non- inflammatory acne as these inhibit the earliest precursor lesions of acne.

In the management of inflammatory acne, these can be used in combination with topical or systemic antimicrobials. These are usually not preferred for nodulocystic acne.

Topical retinoids are most important agents to maintain the favorable results once acne is under control.

Topical therapy of retinoids consists of once-daily application of a thin film of the cream, gel or solution to the entire facial region prone to develop acne lesions. As tretinoin is photolabile, it is to be applied at bedtime. In comparison, adapalene and tazarotene are photostable and can be applied at morning or night.

Side Effects

Topical retinoids may cause skin irritation, including erythema and peeling. This retinoid dermatitis, most problematic during the first few weeks of therapy, is minimized by avoiding harsh soaps, astringents and other irritating agents like scrubs, etc. Alternate-day application (especially early in therapy) and short contact therapy can be suggested if skin irritation is a major concern. Drug holidays, i.e. using drug on weekends is ideal for maintenance therapy.

Tretinoin (All-trans Retinoic Acid; Vitamin A Acid)

Tretinoin is a 1st generation topical retinoid available in 0.025%, 0.05%, 0.1% strength as cream, gel, and lotion. It may cause temporary worsening of acne. It is a category C drug, contraindications include nursing women, pregnancy (relative) and hypersensitivity to the vehicle. Tretinoin should be used cautiously in eczematous skin and sunburn and should not be used simultaneously with BPO as it gets inactivated. It can also have interactions with photosensiti- zing drugs.

Isotretinoin

It is a 2nd generation topical retinoid available in 0.05%, 0.1% cream and 0.05% gel. Isotretinoin loaded with solid lipid nanoparticle formulation does not cause systemic absorption and skin irritation. It does not reduce sebum secretion.

Adapalene

Adapalene is a 3rd generation topical retinoid available as 0.3% and 0.1% gel, cream and microsphere formulation. It is a category C drug whose contraindications include pregnancy (relative) and hypersensitivity to adapalene or the vehicle. It can have interactions with topical sulfur, resorcinol and salicylic acid.

Tazarotene

Tazarotene is a 3rd generation topical retinoid available as 0.1% and 0.05% gel and cream out of which 0.1% is FDA approved for acne. It is a category X drug whose contraindications include pregnancy (absolute) and hypersensitivity to tazarotene or the vehicle. Tazarotene should be used cautiously in eczematous skin and sunburn. It can have interactions with photosensitizing drugs.

Benzoyl Peroxide

Benzoyl peroxide (BPO), a broad-spectrum bactericidal agent, is indicated for the treatment of mild-to-moderate acne vulgaris. It is bactericidal for *P. acnes* (both surface and ductal), inhibits triglyceride hydrolysis, and reduces inflammation in acne lesions.[2] The drug is lipophilic (permitting easy penetration in the pilosebaceous duct) and has keratolytic as well as comedolytic activities.

BPO is available in washes, lotions, creams and gels, ranging from 2.5% to 20%. Approximately 5% of topically applied BPO gets absorbed through the skin and is completely metabolized to benzoic acid which is rapidly cleared by the kidneys without any systemic toxicity. BPO is classified as pregnancy category C drug.

P. acnes has not shown *in vitro* resistance to BPO, making it a useful adjunct for controlling antibiotic resistance and effectively reducing strains of *P. acnes* resistant to antibiotics.

BPO is equally effective as erythromycin or clindamycin on inflammatory lesions, but is more effective on non-inflamed lesions. BPO is comparable to topical tretinoin in management of non-inflammatory lesions but BPO is superior to topical tretinoin for treating inflammatory lesions. BP 4% gel is also comparable to adapalene 0.1% gel in reducing both inflammatory and non-inflammatory lesions.

Side Effects

The major adverse effect of topically applied BPO is irritant dermatitis which causes burning, peeling, erythema and dryness. Water-based gels are less irritating in comparison to alcohol- or acetone-based formulations. Incidence of true contact allergy is 0.2–1%. Patients should be advised that the drug may bleach clothes, hair and other materials.

Topical Antibiotics

Clindamycin, a synthetic derivative of lincomycin (isolated from *Streptomyces* species), is available for topical application as 1% alcohol-based solution, 1% lotion (less irritating) and gel. The drug acts by irreversibly binding to the 50s subunit of the bacterial ribosome, thereby inhibiting bacterial protein synthesis. It is effective against *P. acnes* but an increasing number of clindamycin-resistant strains are associated with treatment failure. Clindamycin is a pregnancy category B drug.

Topical clindamycin is equally effective as or superior to oral tetracycline (in doses up to 1 g/day) for treating inflammatory lesions.[3] Twice-daily application of 1% clindamycin is as effective as oral minocycline 50 mg twice daily. Both 1% clindamycin and 1.5% erythromycin are equally more effective against inflammatory lesions (~60% reduction) than non-inflammatory lesions (~40% reduction).

Side Effects

Mild local reactions (usually due to the vehicle) include burning, stinging, itching, peeling, oily skin, excessive dryness and erythema.[2] Very rarely, clindamycin may cause contact allergy, Gram-negative folliculitis or antibiotic- associated (pseudomembranous) colitis.

Erythromycin

A macrolide antibacterial agent (isolated from *Streptomyces erythreus*), erythromycin is bactericidal through inhibition of bacterial protein synthesis by binding to the 50s subunit of the bacterial ribosome. Topical erythromycin is available in a variety of vehicles in concentrations of 2% and 3%. Erythromycin is classified as pregnancy category B drug.

Erythromycin (1.5–2%) is more effective than placebo for treatment of inflammatory lesions and overall acne grade. In order to circumvent the increasing problem of erythromycin-resistant *P. acnes*, a higher concentration of erythromycin (4%) with or without 1.2% zinc may be used or it can also be used in combination with BPO.

Side Effects

Minor symptoms including burning, itching, irritation, erythema, scaling, tenderness, dryness and oiliness can be seen. Allergic contact dermatitis has been reported infrequently due to erythromycin.

Clarithromycin

It is a macrolide antimicrobial drug (1%) gel for the management of acne and is now withdrawn from the market.

Side Effects

Most common adverse effects include irritation, peeling, redness, stinging and swelling of the skin.

Minocycline

It is tetracycline group of antibiotics. It can be used as a systemic drug in acne. Topical minocycline 4% gel/foam has been approved for inflammatory lesions of non-nodular, moderate to severe acne vulgaris above age of 9 years. It has minimal systemic side effects of minocycline.[3]

Nadifloxacin

It is a fluoroquinolone antibiotic available as 1% cream for the treatment of acne. Nadifloxacin acts by inhibiting DNA gyrase of *P. acnes* which is involved in bacterial DNA synthesis. It also inhibits pro-inflammatory cytokines such as IL-1, IL-6 and IL-8. Nadifloxacin is effective not only against microbial production but also prevents onset of acne scar formation.

Side Effects

Common side effects include erythema, dry skin and peeling.

Dapsone

Dapsone, an antimicrobial and anti-inflammatory agent, is available in a 5% topical gel formulation for the treatment of acne vulgaris. Twice-daily Dapsone 5% gel is effective in reducing non-inflammatory, inflammatory and total lesion counts with greatest reductions occurring in inflammatory lesions. It is classified as pregnancy category C drug.

Side Effects

Most common adverse effects observed are erythema, rash, transient dryness or sunburn. G6PD screening or monitoring of hematologic parameters is not required during treatment with topical dapsone. Topical dapsone has not shown any hypersensitivity reactions.

Sodium Sulfacetamide

Sodium sulfacetamide, commonly incorporated in a formulation with sulfur (a non-specific antifungal/antibacterial), shows anti-inflammatory as well as antibacterial properties, being useful in the treatment of acne.[2] Sulfacetamide inhibits bacterial dihydropteroate synthetase, thereby preventing the conversion of p-aminobenzoic acid (PABA) into folic acid. Sodium sulfacetamide is classified as pregnancy category C drug. Clinical research showed a marked decrease in total acne lesion count and inflammatory lesion count with the use of this drug.

Side Effects

It commonly causes dryness and transient pruritus. If combined with topical preparations containing BPO, sulfacetamide produces an orange-brown discoloration which may stain clothing but not the skin.

Other Drugs

Azelaic Acid

Azelaic acid, available as 10–20% cream and gel, is indicated for the treatment of acne and reduces the concentration of *P. acnes* on the skin surface and follicles in addition to inhibiting the division and differentiation of human keratinocytes, but does not reduce the rate of sebum production. Applying the cream 3–4 times daily can lead to higher penetration into the lesions. Azelaic acid is classified as pregnancy category B drug.

Azelaic acid is comparable with 0.05% tretinoin cream, topical 5% BPO, and topical 2% erythromycin cream in the treatment of mild-to-moderate acne. Azelaic acid also has some role in post-inflammatory hyperpigmentation.[2]

Some patients may report itching, burning or scaling lasting up to a month which can be reduced by initiating treatment with once-daily application during the first few weeks.

Nicotinamide

Nicotinamide, available as 4% gel, has got marked anti-inflammatory properties. It is of comparable efficacy to 1% clindamycin gel in the treatment of acne vulgaris.

Salicylic Acid

It is a topical keratolytic and comedolytic agent, available in 0.5–10% concentration, out of which most commonly used is 2%. It is often used in patients intolerant to topical retinoids.[2] However, it is less comedolytic than tretinoin. Side effects include erythema and peeling.

Sulfur

At lower concentrations, sulfur is thought to have keratoplastic effects and at higher concentrations, a keratolytic effect. However, the therapeutic effect of sulfur in acne may instead be related to non-specific 'irritant' effects that lead to peeling rather than its keratolytic effect.

Sulfur is available as lotion, cream and ointment in concentration 1–10%. Sulfur has been used topically in combination with sodium sulfacetamide (antibacterial agent) in the treatment of acne.[2]

Alpha Hydroxy Acids

These include glycolic acid, lactic acid, glucuronic acid. They reduce the thickness of stratum corneum by decreasing corneocyte adhesion. When used at low concentration (<30%), glycolic acid peels induce epidermal exfoliation and at higher concentrations cause epidermolysis.[2]

Home Remedies

The use of complementary and alternative medications in acne is quite common despite the absence of any evidence- based data on their efficacy, except for a few studies supporting the use of topical tea tree oil.

a. **Tea tree oil:** Due to its anti-inflammatory and anti-bacterial effects, topically applied tea tree oil has a significant effect in reducing the number of inflammatory and non-inflammatory lesions of acne, although the onset of action is slow. A few side effects like dry skin can be experienced.
b. **Green tea:** Topical green tea lotion can be an efficacious and cost-effective treatment for mild-to-moderate acne vulgaris. It may play a role in acne due to the phyto-chemical phenolic compounds. It contains catechins and has antioxidant properties.[3]
c. **Honey:** Since, it has antibacterial properties, it may play a role in the treatment of acne. However, clinical studies proving its efficacy are lacking.
d. **Lemons:** It may act as a skin exfoliant and disinfectant.

Combination Therapy in Acne

Benzoyl peroxide offers the advantage of prevention and elimination of development of *P. acnes* resistance, hence it is being preferred as combination therapy. Its efficacy and tolerability is increased when combined with topical erythromycin/clindamycin.[2] Benzoyl peroxide can also be combined with tretinoin (found to be superior to mono-therapy) but they should not be applied simultaneously as benzoyl peroxide may oxidize tretinoin. Combining a topical retinoid and topical antimicrobial is more effective in reduction of both inflammatory and non-inflammatory lesions in comparison to either agent used alone.

The use of topical BPO—with or without clindamycin—in combination with a topical retinoid represents the standard of care for patients with mild-to-moderate acne vulgaris. The optimized formulation of adapalene and BPO has synergistic benefits early on the reduction of inflammatory/non-inflammatory as well as total acne lesions with rapid onset of efficacy and improved patient adherence due to convenience of therapy.

Topical combination regimens can also be used appropriately in combination with oral acne therapy. Clinical studies have proven that adapalene/BPO gel provides therapeutic benefits when used with oral antibiotics.

Novel Drug Delivery Systems

Encapsulating anti-acne drugs in vesicular/particulate delivery systems represent an innovative and alternative approach in minimizing the side effects and preserving the drug efficacy. Various novel carrier systems under research for management of acne include microsponge, microsphere, microemulsion, liposome, niosome, solid lipid nanoparticles, aerosol, fullerenes, hydrogel, etc. The drug release mechanism of these systems involves diffusion through the carrier matrix, desorption of adsorbed drug, erosion and combination of erosion and diffusion method.

Microsponge Delivery System

Microsponges represent a uniform, spherical and porous polymeric delivery system having a myriad of interconnecting voids within a noncollapsible structure with a large porous surface loaded with the active agent. When applied to the skin, the release of drug can be controlled through diffusion or other variety of triggers, leading to reduced side effects and percutaneous absorption, enhanced product efficacy, mildness and tolerability. They are capable of absorbing skin secretions resulting in reduced oiliness and shine from the skin. It is stable over a wide range of pH and temperature up to 130°C; shows compatibility with most vehicles and ingredients, self-sterilizing (average pore size is 25 µm—impenetrable for bacteria), free flowing and cost effective with a higher payload. Examples include the microsponge of benzoyl peroxide as well as tretinoin, for topical delivery with maintained efficacy and decreased skin irritation/sensitization.

Nanotechnology

A wide range of nanoparticles with different physicochemical properties (polymerised nanoparticles, liposomes, solid lipid nanoparticles), carrying the drug, showed increased follicular penetration, reaching much higher local drug concentrations and optimising the therapeutic effect. A huge advantage of these delivery systems is improved tolerability to irritation caused by retinoids, ultimately resulting in higher patient compliance and prevention of systemic effects from substance absorption. Studies have also shown improved skin tolerance levels and patient satisfaction along with aesthetic attributes after treatment with benzoyl peroxide-microsphere carrier creams.

REFERENCES

1. Liu PT, Krutzik SR, Kim J, Modlin RL. Cutting edge: all-trans retinoic acid down-regulates TLR2 expression and function. The Journal of Immunology. 2005 Mar 1;174(5):2467–70.
2. Leyden JJ, Shalita AR. Rational therapy for acne vulgaris: an update on topical treatment. Journal of the American Academy of Dermatology. 1986 Oct 1;15(4):907–15.
3. Paik J. Topical minocycline foam 4%: a review in acne vulgaris. American Journal of Clinical Dermatology. 2020 Jun;21:449–56.

CHAPTER 12

Newer Treatments in Acne Management

In recent years various newer systemic and topical drugs has been approved and tried in management of acne.

SYSTEMIC DRUGS

COX-2 Inhibitors[1]

Premenstrual acne challenges the conventional therapies of acne. The proposed etiopathogenesis involves female hormones triggering prostaglandins (PGE), particularly PGE 2, initiating acute inflammation in the pilosebaceous unit. Prostaglandins, potent vasoactive substances, are produced locally at inflammation sites.

Mechanism of Action

Cox-2 inhibitors selectively target the enzyme cyclooxygenase 2, hindering PGE2 synthesis with minimal gastrointestinal effects. A study suggests premenstrual dermatological conditions result from hypersensitivity to estrogens and progesterone. Corticosteroids, while effective, pose concerns about prolonged use.

Rofecoxib, a Cox-2 inhibitor, shows promise, albeit with cardiac risks at higher doses. Nonsteroidal anti-inflammatory drugs (NSAIDs), including ibuprofen and benoxaprofen, have been successful in acne treatment. Rofecoxib's once-daily dosage and minimal side effects make it potentially revolutionary in premenstrual acne treatment, suggesting a new era of selective NSAIDs therapy.

Monoclonal Antibodies

The role of interleukin-1 alpha (IL-1α) in comedone formation, activated by *P. acnes* via TLR-2, has spurred innovative approaches in acne therapeutics. Retinoic acid RA-18C3, a monoclonal antibody specific for IL-1α, is currently undergoing phase 2 trials.

Similarly, MABp1 represents the first biologic therapy targeting IL-1α, also in phase 2 trials.[2] Gevokizumab, with its ability to inhibit the IL-1β mediated inflammatory response, is another promising monoclonal antibody in development.[3]

These advancements signify a shift towards targeted immunotherapies, demonstrating the potential of monoclonal antibodies to address specific inflammatory pathways involved in acne pathogenesis.

Vaccines

The role of *P. acnes* CAMP factor in triggering inflammation and cell death underscores its significance in acne vulgaris pathogenesis. Vaccination, particularly targeting CAMP factor 2, emerges as a promising strategy for mitigating *P. acnes*-induced inflammation. The development of a humanized monoclonal antibody (mAb) to CAMP factor holds potential for intralesional therapy, offering a potential alternative to triamcinolone acetonide. Future endeavors should explore the cross-reactivity of antibodies generated by CAMP factor 2 vaccination, paving the way for a multivalent vaccine.[4]

SYSTEMIC DRUGS

Triferotene

Trifarotene is a 4th generation topical retinoids approved on 4 October 2019, by United States (FDA) for the topical treatment of acne vulgaris in patients of 9 years of age and older. It is selective retinoic acid receptor (RAR)-γ agonist employed to treat acne vulgaris on the trunk and face. Because of it's strong selectivity for the skin-predominant RAR-gamma, implying a better local tolerability profile than older generation retinoids, which bind to the other RAR subtypes nonselectively. It is available as 0.005% cream formulation.[5]

Ozenoxacin

Ozenoxacin is a topical quinolone showing potent antimicrobial activities against Gram-negative and Gram-positive bacteria and is widely used for the treatment of inflammatory acne. The production of interleukin (IL)-6 and IL-8 by human epidermal keratinocytes stimulated by heat-killed *Cutibacterium acnes* was significantly inhibited by ozenoxacin. The activation of intracellular pathways, particularly the p38 phosphorylation pathway, was markedly reduced by ozenoxacin in both keratinocytes and THP-1 cells.[6]

Ozenoxacin boasts an exceptional safety profile, with minimal reported adverse effects, making it a reliable choice for dermatological applications. Regarding drug interactions, ozenoxacin's negligible impact on cytochrome P450 enzymes, coupled with minimal systemic absorption, results in a lack of any known drug interactions. The known contraindications include hypersensitivity to the drug or any formulation ingredient.

Clascoterone

Clascoterone is an androgen receptor inhibitor which has been approved for the topical treatment of acne vulgaris in patients 12 years of age and older.[7]

It competes with androgens, especially dihydrotestosterone, for androgen-receptor binding and limits their binding, thus inhibiting downstream signaling of pathways involved in the pathogenesis of acne. It inhibits androgen receptor-regulated gene transcription, and antagonizes lipid and inflammatory cytokine production in a dose-dependent manner in human primary sebocytes. Commercially available as a 1% (10 mg/g) cream, clascoterone exhibits mild and infrequent adverse effects, primarily limited to local skin reactions. Long-term safety assessments highlight its safety, with no systemic antiandrogenic effects observed, such as diminished libido or feminization in male subjects.

Olumacostat Glasaretil (OG): Restraining Fatty Acid Synthesis in Sebaceous Glands

OG intervenes by inhibiting acetyl-coenzyme A carboxylase, the enzyme governing the initial, rate-determining phase of *de novo* fatty acid synthesis. This intervention results in the reduced lipid production of human sebocytes when studied *in vitro*, with the size reduction of sebaceous glands observed *in vivo* in hamster ears. They can thus be indicated as a therapy in patients with moderate to severe acne.[8]

Common AEs were nasopharyngitis, application-site dryness, and application-site pain and application-site erythema.[8]

Stearoyl-coenzyme A Desaturase 1 (SCD-1) Inhibitors

In sebaceous glands SCD-1 is a key enzyme in the synthesis of monounsaturated fatty acids essential for acne development. GSK1940029 gel, a novel SCD-1 inhibitor, is being developed as a potential treatment for acne.[9]

Retinoic Acid Metabolism Blocking Agents (RAMBAs)

It is a novel approach for acne management, with Talarozole emerging as a highly potent and selective azole derivative. It inhibits cytochrome-P450-dependent all-trans-retinoic acid catabolism, it is available in 0.35% and 0.7% gel formulations.

Talarozole's mechanism leads to the normalization of desquamation in the follicular epithelium, effectively reducing comedone formation. This innovative RAMBA contributes to the regulation of skin cell turnover, addressing a key aspect of acne pathogenesis. The development of RAMBAs signifies a promising avenue for refining acne therapeutics and advancing treatments that target specific pathways involved in its development.[10]

Topical Nitric Oxide (NO)

Topical application of NO-releasing nanopeptides exhibits a dual impact on acne, with antimicrobial effects and the suppression of inflammatory cytokines in innate immunity. It effectively suppresses IL-1β, IL-6, IL-8, and TNF-α in human monocytes, along with IL-8 and IL-6 in human keratinocytes. By inhibiting caspase and targeting *P. acnes*, it demonstrates efficacy in phase II trials.

Administered in 1% and 4% concentrations twice daily, the treatment shows statistically significant reductions in both non-inflammatory and inflammatory lesion counts after 12 weeks. This promising approach signifies a potential breakthrough in acne management, addressing both microbial and inflammatory aspects.[11]

Modified Diallyl Disulfide Oxide (M-DDO) and Pirfenidone

The mechanism of action involves direct effects, primarily the inhibition of TNF-α, TGF-β, and other proinflammatory cytokines, mitigating inflammation. Additionally, it modulates Matrix Metalloproteinases (MMPs), preventing scar sequelae. By influencing Keratinocyte Growth Factor (KGF), it regulates keratinocyte production. Its potent antioxidant properties support sebaceous gland metabolism and inhibit inflammatory stimulation by *P. acnes*.

Available in 0.016% gel, cream, and ointment formulations, this antibiotic demonstrates antimicrobial efficacy against both Gram-positive and Gram-negative bacteria. Overall, these advancements contribute to a multifaceted approach to acne treatment, targeting inflammation, scarring, and microbial factors.[12]

Botanical Therapies

Botanical compounds like Epigallocatechin gallate (EGCG), derived from green tea, and Resveratrol, found in grapes and peanuts, offer promising alternatives in acne management. EGCG exhibits anti-inflammatory and sebosuppressive actions, contributing to the reduction of acne-related inflammation and excess sebum production.[12] Similarly, Resveratrol, with its anti-inflammatory properties, plays a sebosuppressive role.

Both compounds, derived from natural sources, provide a botanical approach to acne treatment, addressing key factors in its pathogenesis. These botanical therapies showcase the potential of harnessing plant-derived compounds for their beneficial effects on skin health and may represent a valuable addition to acne treatment strategies.

REFERENCES

1. Tehrani R, Dharmalingam M. Management of premenstrual acne with Cox-2 inhibitors: A placebo controlled study. Indian Journal of Dermatology, Venereology and Leprology. 2004 Nov 1;70:345.
2. Carrasco D, Stecher M, Lefebvre GC, Logan AC, Moy R. An Open Label, Phase 2 Study of MABp1 Monotherapy for the Treatment of Acne Vulgaris and Psychiatric Comorbidity. Journal of Drugs in Dermatology: JDD. 2015 Jun 1;14(6):560–4.

3. Owyang AM, Issafras H, Corbin J, Ahluwalia K, Larsen P, Pongo E, Handa M, Horwitz AH, Roell MK, Haak-Frendscho M, Masat L. XOMA 052, a potent, high-affinity monoclonal antibody for the treatment of IL-1β-mediated diseases. InMAbs 2011 Jan 1 (Vol. 3, No. 1, pp. 49–60). Taylor & Francis.
4. Wang Y, Hata TR, Tong YL, Kao MS, Zouboulis CC, Gallo RL, Huang CM. The anti-inflammatory activities of Propionibacterium acnes CAMP factor-targeted acne vaccines. Journal of Investigative Dermatology. 2018 Nov 1;138(11):2355–64.
5. Naik PP. Trifarotene: a novel therapeutic option for acne. Dermatology Research and Practice. 2022 May 27;2022.
6. Tabara K, Tamura R, Nakamura A, Mori S, Kitano T, Fujikawa K, Fujikawa M, Okamoto K, Kanayama S, Uratsuji H, Ikeda F. Anti-inflammatory effects of ozenoxacin, a topical quinolone antimicrobial agent. The Journal of Antibiotics. 2020 Apr;73(4):247–54.
7. Santhosh P, George M. Clascoterone: a new topical anti-androgen for acne management. International Journal of Dermatology. 2021 Dec;60(12):1561–5.
8. Bissonnette R, Poulin Y, Drew J, Hofland H, Tan J. Olumacostat glasaretil, a novel topical sebum inhibitor, in the treatment of acne vulgaris: A phase IIa, multicenter, randomized, vehicle-controlled study. Journal of the American Academy of Dermatology. 2017 Jan 1;76(1):33–9.
9. Brigandi RA, Zhu J, Murnane AA, Reedy BA, Shakib S. A Phase 1 Randomized, Placebo-Controlled Trial With a Topical Inhibitor of Stearoyl-Coenzyme A Desaturase 1 Under Occluded and Nonoccluded Conditions. Clinical Pharmacology in Drug Development. 2019 Apr;8(3):270–80.
10. Pavez Loriè E, Cools M, Borgers M, Wouters L, Shroot B, Hagforsen E, Törmä H, Vahlquist A. Topical treatment with CYP26 inhibitor talarozole (R115866) dose dependently alters the expression of retinoid-regulated genes in normal human epidermis. British Journal of Dermatology. 2009 Jan 1;160(1):26–36.
11. Baldwin H, Blanco D, McKeever C, Paz N, Vasquez YN, Quiring J, Enloe C, De León E, Stasko N. Results of a phase 2 efficacy and safety study with SB204, an investigational topical nitric oxide-releasing drug for the treatment of acne vulgaris. The Journal of Clinical and Aesthetic Dermatology. 2016 Aug;9(8):12.
12. Yoon JY, Kwon HH, Min SU, Thiboutot DM, Suh. DH. Epigallocatechin-3-gallate improves acne in humans by modulating intracellular molecular targets and inhibiting *P. acnes*. Journal of Investigative Dermatology. 2013 Feb 1;133(2):429–40.

CHAPTER

13

Chemical Peels

For aesthetic management of acne, there are different types of peels available.

INTRODUCTION

Chemical peeling/chemical rejuvenation is a procedure in which peeling agent applied to the skin causing controlled destruction of the layers of the skin at required depth without post peel scarring and pigmentation (Table 13.1).[1]

Mechanism of Action

Chemical peeling is the process of applying chemicals to the skin to destroy the outer damaged layers. The epidermis regenerates from the epidermal appendages located in the remaining dermis. This process begins within 24 hours of wounding and is usually complete in 5–10 days. The new epidermis shows greater organization and vertical polarity, with the disappearance of actinic keratoses and lentigines. Dermal regeneration is a slower process but is usually complete within several months. The regenerated dermis demonstrates less elastosis and improved organization, with compact horizontally arranged bundles of collagen interspersed with elastic fibers. Result is soft supple skin that appears more youthful with fewer rhytides and dyschromias.

Specific Actions

1. It causes inhibition of enzymes like sulfo-transferases, phosphor-transferases, kinase.

Table 13.1: Classification of chemical peels according to depth	
1. **Very superficial light peel** Agents used: TCA 10% GA 30–50% Salicylic acid 20–30% Jessner's solution 1–3 coats Tretinoin 1–5%	Necrosis up to the level of stratum corneum
2. **Superficial peels** Glycolic acid (20–70%) Jessner's solution Salicylic acid Solid CO_2 slush Retinoic acid TCA (10–25%)	Necrosis through the entire epidermis up to basal layer
3. **Medium depth peels** TCA (35–50%) 35% TCA + Jessner's solution 35% TCA + 70% glycolic acid 35% TCA + solid CO_2	Stratum corneum to papillary dermis
4. **Deep peels** Baker-Gordon 88% Phenol >50% TCA	Papillary dermis to upper reticular dermis

Examples: Alpha hydroxyl acids (AHA), retinoic acid, azelaic acid

2. Certain peels cause coagulation of proteins: TCA
3. Enzymatic denaturation and coagulation of proteins: Phenol, resorcinol, salicylic acid

General Guidelines for Peel Procedure

After history taking, doing proper examination to rule out infection any eczematous skin condition, drug intake/allergy.

Proper counseling of the patient about the procedure, results, side effects and post-procedure care is necessary.

Pre- and post-procedure photography under adequate exposure and light for assessment and medicolegal purpose.

Priming: Priming is essential for at least 2–4 weeks prior to the procedure. Priming helps to reduce wound healing time, facilitates uniform penetration of peeling agent, detects intolerance to any agent, enforces patient compliance and reduces the risk of complications.

1. Control any active infection or pre-existing dermatoses.
2. Broad-spectrum sunscreens.
3. Hydroquinone (2–4%) in patients prone to develop post-inflammatory hyperpigmentation.
    a. Patients may also be primed at home by using mild topical peeling agents such as tretinoin 0.025%, adapalene 0.1%, glycolic acid 6–12%, kojic acid, azelaic acid, etc. (agents which are likely to be used in postprocedure maintenance). Tretinoin is known to reduce healing time after resurfacing. The choice of the priming agent depends on the individual physician's preference and individualized patient requirements.
    b. In patients with history of herpes simplex posted for medium depth and deep peels, antiviral therapy with acyclovir or famcyclovir is recommended, beginning two days prior to the procedure and continued for 7–10 days until complete re-epithelialization.

Procedure for Superficial Peels

1. The required strength of the peeling agent is poured into a glass beaker and the neutralizing agent is also kept ready.
2. Sensitive areas like the inner canthus of the eyes and nasolabial folds are protected with Vaseline.
3. The peeling agent is then applied either with a brush or cotton-tipped applicator or gauze.
4. The chemical is applied quickly as cosmetic units on the entire face, beginning from the forehead, then the right cheek, nose, left cheek and chin in that order. If required, the perioral, upper and lower eyelids are treated last. Feathering strokes are applied at the edges to blend with surrounding skin and prevent demarcation lines.
5. For glycolic acid peels, the peel is neutralized after the predetermined duration of time (usually three minutes).

However, if erythema or epidermolysis occurs, seen as grayish white appearance of the epidermis or small blisters, the peel must be neutralized immediately irrespective of the duration. Neutralization is done with 10–15% sodium bicarbonate solution or neutralizing lotion and then, washed off with water.

6. For TCA peels, the end-point is frosting and neutralization is either with a neutralizing agent or cold water, starting from the eyelids and then the entire face.
7. When the salicylic acid peel is applied, it crystallizes forming a pseudo-frost; generally, 1–3 coats are applied to get an even frost. It is then washed with water after 3–5 minutes, after the burning subsides.
8. Jessner's solution is applied in 1–3 coats to get even frosting; the endpoint is erythema or even frosting.
9. A cooling fan helps to reduce burning of the skin.
10. The skin is gently dried with gauze and the patient is asked to wash with cold water until the burning subsides. The face is patted dry; rubbing should be avoided.
11. Tretinoin peels are yellow peels that are left on for 4–5 hours and then washed away.
12. Very superficial peels may be repeated every 1–2 weeks and superficial peels every 2–4 weeks.

ALPHA HYDROXY ACID (AHA) VERSUS BETA HYDROXY ACID (BHA)

These two acid families are considered superficial peels because they only penetrate the outer layer of the skin or the epidermis. They also can treat the same types of skin issues and imperfections such as sun damage, acne scars, smoothing out rough skin and helping the skin appear more youthful, unclog pores and help fight sun damage.

Differences

Alpha hydroxy acids are water soluble while BHAs are oil or lipid soluble (Fig. 13.1). Even though both AHA and BHA only penetrate the outermost layer of the skin (epidermis), because

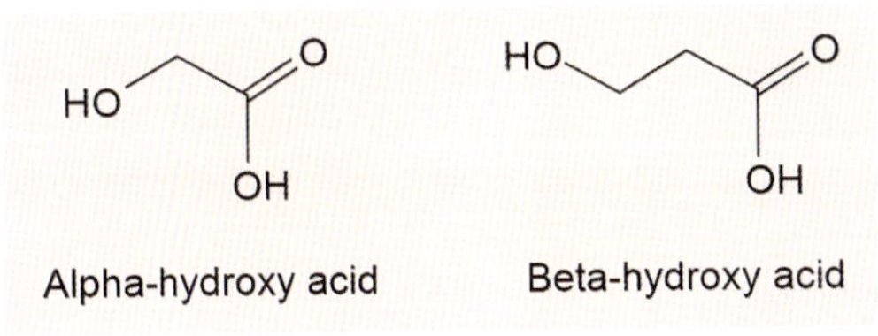

Fig. 13.1: Chemical structure of alpha- and beta-hydroxy acid

BHAs are lipid soluble, they are able to penetrate deeper into the epidermis. BHA has only one acid and that is salicylic acid, while AHAs have several different types, which include: glycolic, lactic, tartaric, malic and citric acids (fruit acids). While both AHA and BHA are used to treat some of the same skin conditions and imperfections, BHA works better for people with sensitive skin and people of colour.

AHA (which is also called glycolic acid) and BHA (also called salicylic acid) are frequently used by physicians to induce light skin peels, which help treat fine lines and wrinkles, acne and uneven texture and coloration. The peel removes a very thin layer of skin, which in turn promotes the growth of new, smoother skin.

SALICYLIC ACID PEEL

Salicylic acid is a beta-hydroxy acid (ortho-hydroxy benzoic acid). Its pKa value is 3. The main difference between alpha-hydroxy acid and beta-hydroxy acid is their lipid solubility. Alpha-hydroxy acids are only water soluble, whereas beta-hydroxy acids are lipid soluble and hence they are capable to penetrate into pores containing sebum and exfoliate dead cells.

Indications

1. Acne (Fig. 13.2)
   - Comedonal acne
   - Inflammatory acne
   - Pigmented acne scars
   - Superficial acne scars
2. Photo aging
   - Fine wrinkles

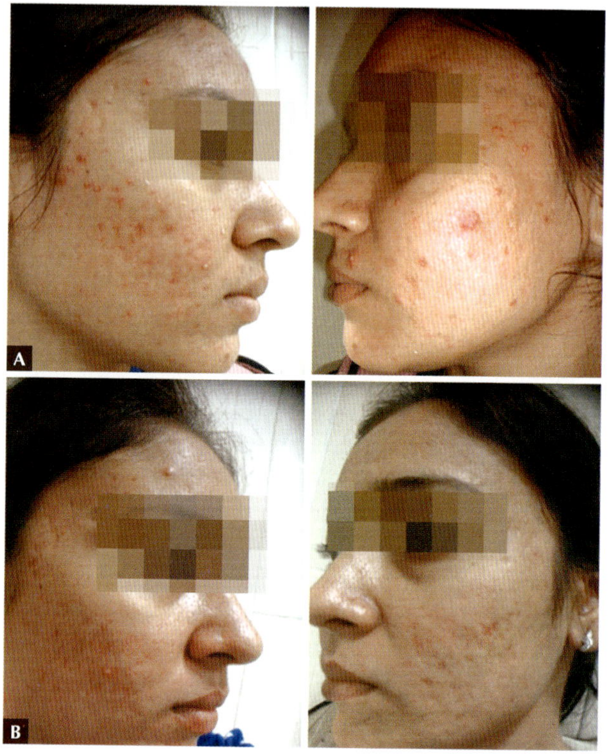

Fig. 13.2: Effect of salicylic acid peel in acne: (A) Baseline; (B) After 6th sitting

3. Textural changes
   - Oily skin
   - Rough uneven skin
   - Dilated pores
4. Acne rosacea

Contraindications

Any allergy to salicylates/aspirin, pregnancy, lactation, unrealistic patient expectations, dermatitis at peeling site, excessively dry skin, patient on isotretinoin.

Peel Procedure

Salicylic acid 20% peel is quickly applied in two to three coats to get a uniform peel. Patient will experience a stinging and burning sensation which increases over the next 2 minutes, reaches a peak and then rapidly decreases to baseline over the next minute.

Pseudofrost develops because of evaporation of hydroethanolic vehicle, not due to protein coagulation. This appears at about 30 sec to 1 min after applying the peeling agent. If there is an uneven area of SA frost, the peel is reapplied in that area. The penetration of the active agent stops once the vehicle has volatilized. At this point, there is no burning or stinging. The patient is instructed to wash the face with cold water and pat the face dry. Postpeel care is advised as in any other peel.

Complications

Crusting, desquamation, inflammation and erythema can occur. Moisturizers, topical steroid cream like hydrocortisone 1% can be used in case of any side effects.

GLYCOLIC ACID PEELS

Biochemistry

It is alpha-hydroxy acid. One hydroxyl group is attached to the alpha position of the carboxyl group. Both this group are attached to aliphatic or aromatic carbon chain. Acidic property is due to carboxyl group. It is fruit acid, extracted from sugarcane. It is hydrophilic acid. Activity or acidifying power of glycolic acid peel is determined by pH of the solution. Between 35 and 70% concentration it is used as peeling agent.

Mechanism of Action

It causes controlled chemical burn of the skin by its dual mode of action. At low concentration and pH it causes breakage of corneodesmosomes by inhibiting enzymes kinases, sulfo-transferases, phosphotransferases which are responsible for cohesion of corneocytes. It does not cause coagulation of proteins, hence there is no frosting seen. The greyish discoloration seen with higher concentrations is due to epidermolysis and a sign of over peeling. Since they do not bind with proteins, they are not self-neutralizing like TCA and have to be neutralized to stop their action. The contact time of the acid with the skin is important as greater the contact time, deeper is the peel.

There is stimulation of growth in basal layers of epidermis and they try to restore optimum barrier function as soon as possible. In the dermis it cause synthesis of collagen, elastin, glycosaminoglycan. It decreases melanin production by direct inhibition of tyrosinase enzyme.[2,3]

Indications

Comedonal acne, post-acne pigmentation, superficial scarring and dilated pores.

Contraindications

Active viral, fungal, bacterial infection particularly herpes. Seborrheic dermatitis, contact dermatitis, atopic dermatitis. Patients on photosensitizing drugs.

One who had deep resurfacing procedure like dermabrasion, laser surgery. Uncooperative patients or patients with unrealistic expectation.

Contact Time

Natural pH of an aqueous solution of 60% glycolic acid is 0.5. Very superficial (upper epidermis): 25–50% partially buffered, for 1–2 mins

- Superficial (papillary dermis): 50–70% partially buffered, for 2–10 mins.
- Medium depth (mid-deep dermis): 70% unbuffered, for 5–10 mins. Not recommended in colored skin.

On the face, a 50% concentration for 1–3 mins is effective, whereas for the back a 70% concentration for 4–8 mins is required.

Contact time should gradually be prolonged by 30–60 seconds for subsequent sessions.

Peel Procedure

Ask the patient to wash face with soap and water. Skin is disinfected with alcohol, degreased with acetone (pre-peel cleanser). Patient should be seated or lying down at 45° and hair pulled back with hair band. Sensitive areas like inner and outer canthus of eye, nasal crease protected with Vaseline. Glycolic acid solution should be applied quickly around 15–20 seconds so that contact time remain same for whole face. A faint erythema is endpoint. It is difficult in dark skin people to appreciate which sometimes results in postinflammatory hyperpigmentation. If endpoint exceeded epidermolysis occurs, seen as whitening and blistering.

Postprocedure Care

A good postprocedure care system is essential to reduce the risk of potential complications and ensure early recovery of normal skin. The postprocedure care depends on the condition being treated. The barrier function of the skin is impaired after a glycolic acid peel. Sunscreens are essential to prevent erythema and PIH, particularly in darker skins. If there is excessive desquamation, a non-occlusive water based moisturizer should be applied to reduce discomfort and excessive picking of the skin, which can delay healing. The peels can be repeated every 2 weeks initially till a satisfactory response is obtained. Thereafter, maintenance peels may be required particularly for photoaging and melasma.

TRICHLOROACETIC ACID

Trichloroacetic acid is a strong acid with pKa 0.26. It is used for superficial as well as medium depth peels. It has a caustic action and causes coagulation of proteins. TCA gets neutralized by the serum in deep dermal vasculature, so it does not require a specific neutralizer. The depth of destruction depends on the concentration of TCA. The higher the concentration, the deeper is the penetration; hence it has a predictable effect. Coagulation is followed by inflammation and activation of mechanisms of wound repair. This leads to re-epithelialization with replacement of smoother skin with an even skin tone. Medium depth peels cause collagen remodelling, with production of new collagen in the dermis. It is available as anhydrous, hygroscopic white crystals, which are dissolved in distilled water to make solution. It should be stored in glass bottle. Now commercial preparations are available.

Superficial TCA peel: 10%, 20%, 25% concentration Deep TCA peel: Above 35%.

Superficial TCA peels are available in 10%, 20%, 25% concentration.

Deep TCA peels are with concentration above 35%.

Indications[4]

1. Photoaging
   - Fine wrinkles
2. Textural changes
   - Oily skin
   - Rough uneven skin
   - Dilated pores
3. Acne
   - Pigmented acne scars
   - Superficial mild acne scars

Contraindications

Medium depth peels should be avoided in patients with keloidal tendency, atrophic skin or recent facial surgical procedures, within the last 6 months such as resurfacing, grafts, flaps, etc. which may have compromised circulation and delayed healing.

Procedure

Very superficial peel-no frosting or very minute speckles of frost superficial peel-scattered frosting with mild erythema is seen (Level 1). A superficial full thickness epidermal peel is achieved by a second coat to get a speckled whiter frost with erythema showing through deeper medium depth peel up to papillary dermis. A solid white frost seen, should be avoided.

Complication

Pigmentation is a common complication in dark skinned patient. The deeper the peel, the greater is the risk of complications. Medium depth peel can be associated with complications like persistent erythema, hyper- or hypopigmentation, scarring, milia, delayed healing, textural changes.

JESSNER'S PEEL

Jessner's peel is a combination of an alpha-hydroxy acid lactic acid and a beta-hydroxy acid. Salicylic acid along with a phenol derivative resorcinol in alcohol. In a modified Jessner's peel, resorcinol has been replaced by citric acid.

Jessner's peel (Combe's peel)	*Modified Jessner's peel*
Lactic acid 14%	Lactic acid 17%
Salicylic acid 14 gm	Salicylic acid 17 gm
Resorcinol 14 gm	Citric acid 8%
Ethanol to make	Ethanol to make
100 ml	100 ml

Indications

- Acne vulgaris
- Superficial acne scars
- Dilated pores

Contraindications

Contraindications are allergy to resorcinol, salicylates other than regular contraindications for chemical peel.

Procedure

Jessner's solution is applied in one to three coats till even Frosting appears. The endpoint is erythema or even frosting. No neutralization is needed. Ice cold compresses may be given after washing the face with cold water.

Complications

Complications are rare as Jessner's peels are superficial peels. Allergic reactions may occur to resorcinol or salicylic acid. Allergy to resorcinol can manifest as pruritus, erythema and disproportionate edema, 5–7 days after a peel. Systemic toxicity can occur with both resorcinol and salicylic acid when used over large areas.

LACTIC ACID PEEL

Biochemistry

Lactic acid (2-hydroxypropanoic acid) is a mild alpha-hydroxy acid (AHA) derived from sour milk, bilberries, yogurt and tomato juice. Lactic acid is a natural constituent found in muscle fiber. At a lower pH (less than 3.5) and in high concentrations, lactic acid acts as a peeling agent. It is also a component of Jessner's peel along with salicylic acid and resorcinol. It has also been used in combination peels with other peeling agents in varying concentrations.

Mechanism of Action

Lactic acid has antimicrobial and anti-inflammatory properties. It acts by dissolving the intercellular desmosomes to promote desquamation of the stratum corneum. It is also said to increase the hyaluronic acid content in the skin and act as a part of skin's natural moisturizing factor. Hence, it improves skin texture and smoothen the skin. Like any AHA, it can also reverse photo damage and reduce wrinkles, brown spots. It has a comparatively large molecule which allows it to penetrate slowly, thus decreased chances of treatment- induced inflammation and irritation.

Indications

- Dry or dehydrated skin
- Melasma
- Superficial atrophic acne scars

Advantages

Lactic acid has the largest molecular weight among AHAs, penetration is much slower which results in less irritation to the skin. It can be safely used in patients with sensitive skin and in patients with rosacea. As lactic acid is a humectant, it can also be used in patients with dry mature skin. It is a safe peel to perform on patients who are new to peels. Lactic acid acts as an exfoliator and moisturizer by removing the outer layers of thickened damaged skin thus providing a smoother appearance. It has also been useful in improving the barrier function of the skin. Since it is naturally occurring in the skin, allergic reactions are rare.

Disadvantages

It is less effective alone as a peeling agent, better results are obtained in combination with other peels. It is a good moisturizing agent, beneficial in dry skin conditions.

MANDELIC ACID

Also known as 'German mandel-almond', which is a natural AHA, which can be obtained from amygdalin, a glycoside found in bitter almonds, peaches and apricots. This AHA contains a phenyl group as a side chain substituent. This changes the solubility profile of the AHA, rendering it more lipophilic compared to other conventional water-soluble.

AHAs and hence can be used to treat oily and acne-prone skin.

Mechanism of Action

Mandelic acid possesses antiseborrheic and keratolytic properties. It is also known to stimulate collagen synthesis and inhibit melanogenesis. Mandelic acid is partially soluble in water and freely soluble in isopropyl and ethyl alcohol.

Mandelic acid has a pKa of 3.41 and is stronger than glycolic acid which has a pKa of 3.83 at 25°C. Higher concentrations of 20%, 40% and 50% are used as peeling agents. Lower concentrations of 2% are used as a face wash and 2–10% for home use.[6]

Indications

- Photodamage
- Acne

Procedure

The peel is usually applied for 5 minutes or longer depending on the patient's skin condition. It may even be left for 12 hours after which it is gently washed off. The peel is usually repeated in 2 weeks and about 6–8 sessions are required to get good cosmetic results.

Advantages

Mandelic acid has anti-aging properties hence it is useful for rejuvenating the skin and improving skin texture. It also has antibacterial properties; hence it is useful for acne.

PYRUVIC ACID

Pyruvic acid (CH_3-CO-COOH) is an alpha-keto acid that is converted under physiological conditions to lactic acid;

the corresponding AHA which is one of the most effective natural humectants for human skin. The effect of pyruvic acid depends on the concentration used and the duration of application before neutralization. It is a potent acid due to its low pKa of 2.39 and has a small molecule allowing deeper penetration.[7]

Mechanism of Action

Pyruvic acid has the keratolytic action of an alpha-keto acid and the humectant effect of lactic acid, combination of which makes it an effective peeling agent. At the epidermal level pyruvic acid induces keratinocytes detachment, epidermolysis and thinning of the upper epidermal layers. At the dermal level, pyruvic acid causes an increase in production of collagen, elastic fibers and glycoproteins. Pyruvic acid also has sebostatic and antimicrobial activities.[8] Pyruvic acid is well suited for treating oily skin and acne because of its lipophilic nature.

Indications

- Acne
- Seborrhea

Procedure

After cleansing and degreasing the skin, pyruvic acid is applied with a gauze and rubbed gently until erythema appears. There is a burning and stinging sensation which reduces after neutralizing with a solution containing 10% sodium bicarbonate in water. Erythema generally persists for a few hours. Mild desquamation occurs for 7–10 days after peeling.

COMBINATION PEEL

Combination Peels and Procedures

Combination of peeling agents enhances the depth of the peel without using a higher concentration of the peeling agent. However, these medium depth peels should be used cautiously in darker skinned patients because of the risk of uneven depth of peeling and increased risk of side effects, such as postinflammatory hyperpigmentation and scarring.

1. Glycolic acid 70% combined with TCA 35% (Coleman's peel). In darker skins, lower concentrations of TCA (10– 25%) may be used.
2. Solid CO_2 combined with 35% TCA (Brody's peel).
3. Jessner's solution with 35% TCA (Monheit's peel).

Two procedures can also be combined to blend cosmetic units and avoid demarcation lines:

1. Chemical peeling combined with dermabrasion: This procedure was originally used by combining application of 50% TCA followed by dermabrasion for post-acne scarring. However, 50% TCA causes scarring and its use is not advocated anymore.
2. Chemical peeling can also be combined with laser resurfacing for skin rejuvenation. First, a chemical peel is performed and then the deeper wrinkles in the periorbital and perioral areas are treated with pulsed CO_2 laser (level C).
3. Chemical peel with dermasanding using sandpaper (level C).
4. Chemical peeling with botulinum toxin (level C).
5. Chemical peeling with fillers (level C).

Coleman Version Glycolic Acid and Trichloracetic Acid Peel[9]

The combination of glycolic acid 70% and trichloracetic acid 35% is another combined peel designed to improve the efficacy of 35% trichloracetic acid without the risks and complications of higher strength TCA. Chemicals, methodology and techniques are different so that one must have a thorough understanding of this peel and not utilize the methods of the preceding combination peel or the use of trichloracetic acid alone. This combination peel produces less wounding depth, but a significantly greater wound level than 35% trichloracetic acid alone. It has also demonstrated the ability to stimulate new collagen production with a comparable Grenz zone to the other medium depth peels. Application of the glycolic acid prior to the TCA peel allows for an even debridement of the stratum corneum equal to that obtained with a degreasing procedure and the Jessner's solution.

In this procedure, no cleansing or degreasing procedure is done. After washing the face with soap and water, 70% glycolic acid is applied directly to the patient's facial skin with swab and after a strict 2 minute contact period, the solution is removed with tap water. Next, the 35% trichloracetic acid is applied in a sequential pattern with either cotton tip applicators or 4 × 4 inch gauze pads to the entire face. The usual frosting is obtained and cool compresses are placed to alleviate the stinging and burning.

This combination peel has also been found effective in the treatment of actinic keratoses and epidermal growths, Glogau grade II photoaging skin, and pigmentary dyschromias. The same skin preparations are used as well as similar postoperative wound care.

Drawbacks may be the uneven nature of glycolic acid peeling and the possibility of accentuating "TCA hot spots." In addition, the use of saline to neutralize the glycolic acid may inhibit some of the absorption of trichloracetic acid for the second part of this combination peel.

Other medium depth peels include:[10]

- Full strength unoccluded phenol peel.
- Pyruvic acid (alpha-keto acid).
- Jessner's-glycolic acid peel.

Eighty-nine percent phenol has the ability to wound through the papillary dermis similar to other peeling strengths discussed. Its disadvantage is inherent in the absorption of phenol with significant cardiac and hepatorenal toxicity. For this reason, the other peels discussed have significant advantages.

Pyruvic acid is an alpha-keto acid which is a very potent chemical peeling agent and has been used experimentally for photoaging skin. The rapid dermal penetration has the potential for scarring and side effects and though some results have been demonstrated by Griffin to be excellent, its safety and efficacy has not been well established.

Jessner's Solution and Glycolic Acid Peel

This combination peel has been studied with the intent of two theoretical advantages.

- Jessner's solution allows for deeper penetration of the glycolic acid.

- The glycolic acid will be a greater stimulant for collagen regeneration without further exfoliation. Though this technique is both time-dependent and restricted to visual endpoints, the chances for over treating are great which may create potential side effects and complications.

JESSNER'S TCA PEEL

It is a method of chemoexfoliation, a combination of two acidic compounds. It is effective in medium depth peel for photo-ageing skin, actinic keratosis and rhytides.[10]

The Jessner's TCA peel procedure is as follows:

1. The skin should be cleaned thoroughly with Septisol® to remove oils.
2. Acetone or acetone alcohol is used to further debride oil and scale from the surface of the skin.
3. Jessner's solution is applied.
4. Thirty-five percent TCA is applied until a light frost appears.
5. Cool saline compresses are applied to dilute the solution.
6. The peel will heal with 0.25% acetic acid soaks and a mild emollient cream.

There is an immediate burning sensation as the peel solution is applied, but this subsides as frosting is completed. Cool saline compresses offer symptomatic relief for a peeled area as the solution is applied to other areas.

Postoperatively, edema, erythema, and desquamation are expected. With periorbital peels and even forehead peels, eyelid edema can occur and may be enough to close the lids. For the first 24 hours, the patient is instructed to soak four times a day with a 0.25% acetic acid compress made of 1 tablespoon white vinegar in 1 pint of warm water. A bland emollient is applied to the desquamating areas after soaks. After 24 hours, the patient can shower and clean gently with a mild nondetergent cleanser. The erythema intensifies as desquamation becomes complete within 4–5 days. Thus, healing is completed within 1 week to 10 days. At the end of 1 week, the bright red color has faded to pink and has the appearance of a sun burn. This can be covered by cosmetics and will fade fully within 2–3 weeks.

The medium-depth peel is dependent on three components for therapeutic effect:

1. Degreasing
2. Jessner's solution, and
3. 35% TCA.

The amount of each agent applied creates the intensity and thus the effectiveness of this peel. The variables can be adjusted according to the patient's skin type and the areas of the face being treated.

Tretinoin and Retinol Peels

Tretinoin and retinol peels have become popular peeling agents because of the favorable results shown by their use in a few of the recent studies. The other reasons for their popularity are ease of application, lack of burning sensation and patient satisfaction. They offer predictable depth control and produce superficial exfoliation. They are considered safe, with a low incidence of side effects.

The retinoid family comprises vitamin A (retinol) and its natural derivatives such as retinaldehyde, retinoic acid and retinyl esters, as well as a large number of synthetic derivatives Retinol is a 20-carbon molecule that consists of a cyclohexenyl ring side chain with four double bonds (all in trans configuration) and an alcohol end group, hence the name all-trans retinol.

Mode of Action

Tretinoin activates three nuclear retinoic acid receptors (RAR-alpha, RAR-beta and RAR-gamma), which bind to regulatory regions in DNA and activate many gene transcriptions. This is responsible for the various epidermal and dermal changes seen with retinoids (Table 13.2).

Indications

- Photoaging: Solar lentigines, dullness and rough skin texture.
- Fine lines
- Enlarged pores
- Melasma
- Ephelides

Table 13.2: Epidermal and dermal changes seen with retinoids[11–13]

Mechanism of action	*Clinical effects*
Epidermal changes • Cellular differentiation • Compaction of stratum corneum • Epidermal hyperplasia	Improvement in texture : Increased smoothness and reduced roughness
Melanin dispersion	Improvement in pigmentation
Collagen stimulation	Reduction in fine wrinkles Improvement in atrophy

- Post-inflammatory hyperpigmentation
- Comedonal acne and papulopustular acne
- Acne-induced pigmentation

Peel Technique

Solutions: The peel solution is applied to the least reactive areas first, such as the forehead, then the periphery of the cheeks, followed by nose, upper lip, chin and then to the more sensitive areas such as the medial face. Open bottles or soaked applicators should never be passed over the patient's eyes.

Creams: The cream formulation is applied using gloved hands in a single layer. A coin-sized amount of retinol cream is dispensed onto a gloved hand. An equal-sized amount is placed in 4 quadrants of the face, namely, forehead, bilateral cheeks and medial face (nose, upper lip and chin). The cream is spread and lightly massaged using fingertips in small circular motions. A using fingertips is applied along the jawline to feather the edges of the treatment area. The cream is continued to be massaged until it is absorbed and almost dried. The skin feels slightly tacky and shows a yellow discoloration.

Termination: Retinoid peels are self-neutralizing and therefore do not require application of a neutralizing agent. The peel is left on the skin and patient is instructed to wash the face at home after 4–8 hours with a gentle cleanser. However, if excessive irritation occurs such as excessive burning, vesiculation or whitening of the skin, then the peel is terminated by removing the peel product using a dry gauze.

Complications: Retinoid peels generally have a very low-risk of untoward complications. Occasionally, they can occur.

- Burning sensation
- Transient hyperpigmentation
- Prolonged erythema
- Excessive scaling in localized areas, such as the cheeks, eyelids and the perioral region.
- Contact dermatitis
- Vesiculation
- Infection
- Acne exacerbation
- Herpes simplex activation.

BLACK PEEL

Black peel is a new chemical peel solution based on black vinegar (black acetic acid).

Ingredients

Tetra-hydro-jasmonic acid and salicylic acid: Plays an important role in the pathogen defense response, have anti-inflammatory effect as well as exfoliating property.

Potassium iodide: Empirically used for deep fungal infection and has wound recovery effect.

Black acetic acid: Contains large amount of organic materials, minerals and especially high concentrations of essential amino acids. It has anticancer properties as well as antioxidant activity.

Indications

- **Acne:** Pustules, nodules-black peel clear and black peel spot
- Improves PIH.
- Skin resurfacing, cell renewal, anti-oxidant-black peel resurfacing.

Black Peel Procedure

Step 1: Preparation-cleanser and toner.

Step 2: Comedones extraction.

Step 3: Application of black peel clear—Apply this solution starting from the outside edges of the face, leaving the sensitive areas of the face until the last moment. Apply the solution two times or more on the oozing or bleeding acne lesions opened by extraction. Wait approximately 10 minutes to calm down the redness and warming sensation. Cleanse with the soft sponge soaked in cold water.

Step 4: Sebo Hydra Infused Mask—Apply mask on the face to calm down and hydrate the irritated skin. For deeper penetration, use Sonophoresis for 5–10 minutes and leave it for another 10 minutes. Do not rinse after taking it off, instead, massage gently the residue to be absorbed completely.

Step 5: Sunscreen.

Black Peel Protocol

Day 0: Black peel application at office.

Day 1–5: Peeling occurs.

Day 6–13: *Black peel acne spot (home care):* Contains black acetic acid, bio sulfur (comedolytic), potassium iodide, jasmonic acid, salicylic acid and lactic acid. Patient applies at home over black and white heads, nodules, cysts and pores several times for maximum penetration and leaves overnight.

Day 14–20: Time for healing.

Day 21: Black peel.

Four to six sessions are recommended depending on acne severity.[11]

REFERENCES

1. Khunger N. Basics of chemical peeling. In: Khunger N (Ed). Step by Step Chemical Peels, 1st edition. New Delhi: Jaypee Brothers; 2009;7–17.
2. Khunger N. Glycolic acid peels. In: Khunger N (Ed). Step by Step Chemical Peels, 1st edition. New Delhi: Jaypee Brothers; 2009; 69–87.
3. M. Salicylic acid peels. Indian J Dermatol Venereol Leprol. 2004; 70:136–8.

4. Savant SS. Superficial and medium depth chemical peeling. In: Savant SS (Ed). Textbook of Dermatosurgery and Cosmetology, 2nd edition. ASCAD, 2005;177-95.
5. Khunger N (Ed). Step by Step Chemical Peels, 1st edition. New Delhi: Jaypee Medical Publishers; 2009. pp. 90,96,140–1,150– 2,156.
6. Khunger N. Step by Step Chemical Peels, 1st Edition. New Delhi: Jaypee Brothers Medical Publishers; 2009. pp. 36, 52, 53, 141, 161, 162, 202–05, 211–18, 280–97.
7. Garg VK, Sinha S, Sarkar R. Glycolic acid peels versus salicylic-mandelic acid peels in active acne vulgaris and post-acne scarring and hyperpigmentation: a comparative study. Dermatol Surg. 2009;35:59–65.
8. Cotellessa C, Manunta T, Ghersetich I, et al. The use of pyruvic acid in the treatment of acne. J Eur Acad Dermatol Venereol. 2004;18:275–8.
9. The glycolic acid trichloroacetic acid peel, Coleman WP 3rd, Futrell JM., J Dermatol Surg Oncol. 1994 Jan; 20(1):76–80. PMID:8288810.
10. Brody HJ. Chemical peeling and resurfacing. Mosby, St Louis; 1997:109–110. The Journal of Dermatologic Surgery and Oncology 15(9):945–50.
11. Sarkar R, Roberts WE, Ghunawat S, Mandlewala ZK, Aggarwal I. Chemical Peels: A Global Perspective. Jaypee Brothers Medical Publishers; 2019 Aug 31.
12. Darlenski R, Surber C, Fluhr JW. Topical retinoids in the management of photodamaged skin: from theory to evidence-based practical approach. British Journal of Dermatology. 2010 Dec 1;163(6):1157–65.
13. Baldwin HE, Nighland M, Kendall C, Mays DA, Grossman R, Newburger J. 40 years of topical tretinoin use in review. Journal of Drugs in Dermatology: JDD. 2013 Jun 1;12(6):638–42.

CHAPTER 14

Acne Scar

INTRODUCTION

A scar is a fibrous tissue that develops as a result of healing at the site of a previous wound or trauma. Cutaneous scarring is a macroscopic defect of the normal structure and function of the skin which represents itself as a raised or depressed area, with an altered skin texture, appearance, color, vascularity, nerve supply and biomechanical properties.

Acne vulgaris is a chronic inflammatory disorder of the pilosebaceous unit, which usually manifests in adolescence with pleomorphic lesions like comedones, papule, pustules, nodules, cysts which may get infected. Scarring is a well- known complication of acne vulgaris.

One of the most common consequences of acne are the scars which are quite disturbing. Features which are important in development of acne scars are:

- Severity of acne.
- Delay in starting an adequate treatment.
- Even grade 1 acne can scar.

PATHOGENESIS OF ACNE SCARRING

Injury to the normal skin initiates a complex process of physiological wound healing which is:

a. Inflammation.
b. Granulation tissue formation (proliferation).
c. Remodeling of matrix tissue (maturation)

Acne scars result from an abnormal response to wound healing at various stages.

Inflammation

The process of inflammation in acne is localized to the pilosebaceous units of skin. Proliferation of *Propionibacterium acnes* lead to stimulation of the innate immune response and activation of complement components leading to inflammation and cytokine release.[1, 2] The appearance of a scar correlates to the extent and depth of inflammation. With the dermal involvement, there is an extensive degradation of the dermal matrix, hence leading to scarring.[3]

Melanin production is also stimulated during inflammation. Hence, it is important for development of post-acne pigmentation and erythema.

Proliferation Phase

Fibroblasts from dermis migrate into the wound in order to synthesize the reparative tissue: The extracellular matrix. Granulation tissue is made by procollagen, elastin, proteoglycans and hyaluronic acid. Particular members of fibroblasts called myofibroblast that make actin filaments are responsible for wound contraction.

The composition of immature scar is predominantly made up of type III collagen, with a small percentage (20%) of type I collagen. There is a shift in the collagen type in mature scars which mimics normal unwounded skin, with approximately 80% of type I collagen.[4]

Remodelling of Matrix Tissue

After healing of the wound, the immature scar passes into final maturation phase, which nearly lasts for a few months. This multistep process is regulated by several molecules including epidermal growth factor (EGF), basic fibroblast growth factor (bFGF), transforming growth factor-beta (TGF-β), mitogen activated protein kinases (MAPs), matrix metalloproteinases (MMPs).

Matrix metalloproteinases (MMPs) are extracellular matrix (ECM) degrading enzymes that form a pathway for remodeling of the ECM. Activation of NF-κB and activator protein-1 (AP-1) leads to upregulation of MMPs like MMP-1, MMP-8, MMP-9 and MMP-13. These are involved in degradation of collagen. The pathway of upregulation of MMPs and procollagen synthesis are prolonged in acne scar prone patients.[5] There is imbalance in the ratio of MMPs to tissue inhibitors of MMPs which result in the development of atrophic or hypertrophic scar (Fig. 14.1).[6] For example, increase in levels of MMP-2 and decrease in levels of MMP-9 are found in hypertrophic and keloid scars causing lack and/or late apoptotic death of myofibroblasts, hence fibrogenesis is prolonged.

The degree of severity of the scar depends on depth and extent of inflammation. If only epidermis and superficial dermis are involved, scar may appear as erythematous or hyperchromic macule. If deep dermis is affected, sharp walled or ice-pick scars are produced. If more extensive deep dermal damage

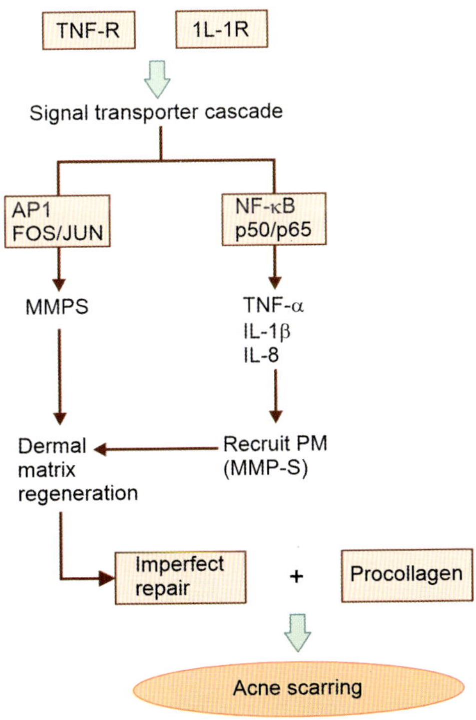

Fig. 14.1: A hypothetical model of pathophysiology of inflammatory acne and dermal damage leading to scarring.[5]

occurs, broad scars can develop like rolling scars or boxcar scars. Follicular and perifollicular acne inflammation induces hypopigmented scars.

In acne patients not prone to scar, the time course was typical of a type IV delayed hypersensitivity response, effective resolution occurred by both non-specific/innate and adaptive immune mechanisms. In lesions from acne patients who were prone to scar, a predominantly adaptive immune response was present, which was persistent and up-regulated in resolving lesions. This suggests that effective management of inflammation during the development and resolution stages of acne may help to control scarring.[7]

CLASSIFICATION

Either a result of increased or lack of tissue formation, acne scars may be classified as (Figs 14.2 and 14.3):

1. Atrophic scars
2. Hypertrophic scars

Atrophic Acne Scars

Atrophic acne scars are more common than hypertrophic scars.

The ratio is 3:1. Atrophic scars can be classified into three types:

Ice-pick scars: Narrow (<2 mm in diameter), deep, sharply marginated, and depressed track that extends vertically into deep dermis and subcutaneous tissue. The opening is usually wider than the deeper infundibulum as the scar tapers from the surface to its deepest apex, hence forming a V-shape (Fig. 14.4).

Boxcar scars: Round to oval depressions with sharply demarcated vertical edge. These are wider at surface and do not taper to a point at base. These scars may be shallow (0.1–0.5 mm) or deep (>0.5 mm) and diameter may vary from 1.5 mm to 4.0 mm. These are U-shaped scars.

Rolling scars: These occur from dermal tethering of otherwise normal-appearing skin and are usually wider than 4–5 mm in diameter. An abnormal fibrous anchoring of the dermis to the

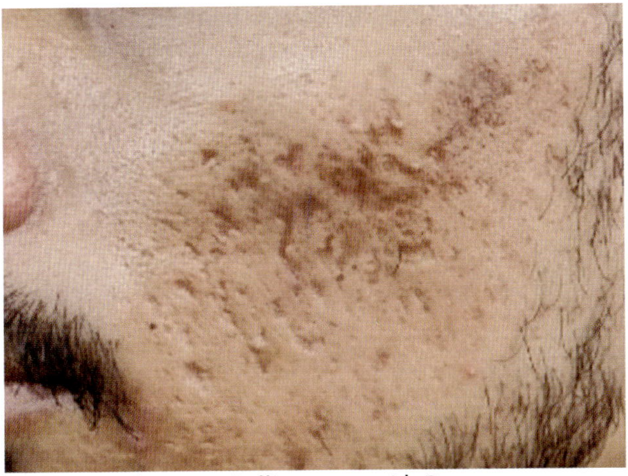

Fig. 14.2: Rolling scars with Boxcars

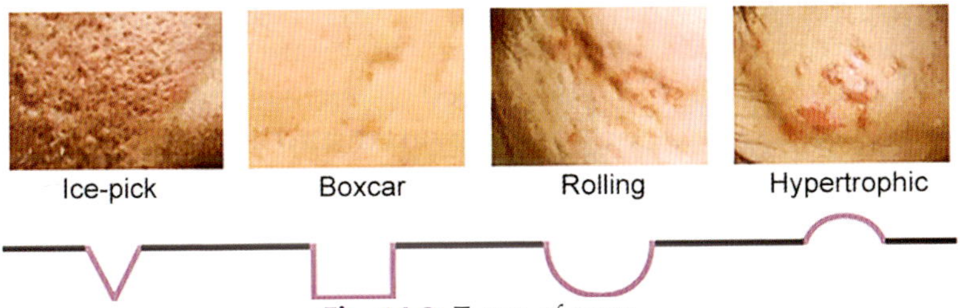

Fig. 14.3: Types of scars

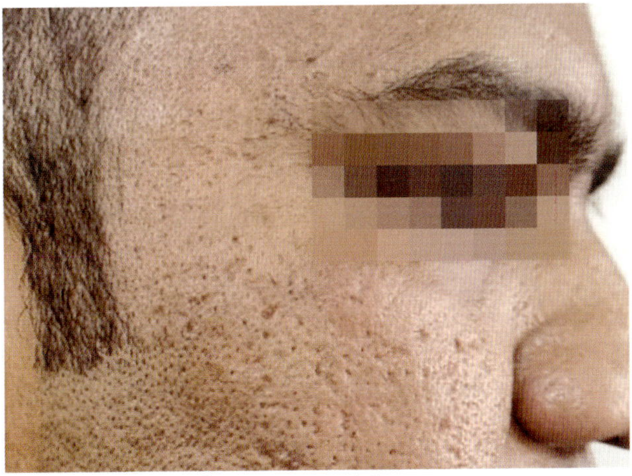

Fig. 14.4: Ice-pick scars

subcutaneous tissue leads to superficial shadowing and to a rolling or undulating appearance of overlying skin.

Amongst atrophic scars, the ice pick type represents 60–70% of total scars, the boxcar 20–30% and rolling scars 15–25%.

Atrophic Macules

These are soft, often with a slightly wrinkled base, and may be bluish in appearance due to blood vessels lying just under the scar.

Follicular Macular Atrophy

These are small, white, soft lesions, often barely raised above the surface of the skin.

Hypertrophic Scars

Hypertrophic and keloidal scars are associated with increase in collagen deposition and decreased collagenase activity.

Hypertrophic scars are elevated and firm with thick hyalinized collagen bundles. These remain within the borders of the original site of injury (Fig. 14.5).

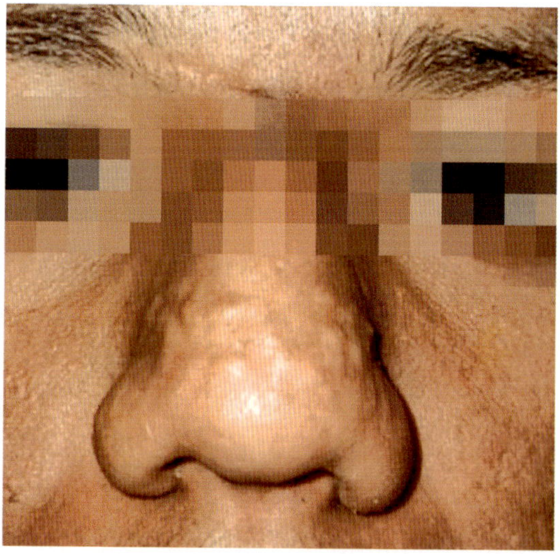

Fig. 14.5: Hypertrophic (popular) scars over nose

Keloids form as reddish-purple papules and nodules that extend beyond the borders of the original wound. Histologically, these are characterized by thick bundles of hyalinised acellular collagen arranged in whorls.

Hypertrophic acne scars and acne-associated keloids occur predominantly on the torso (upper and mid-aspect of back, sternum and clavicular areas, shoulders and deltoids, and occasionally over the jaw angles).

Sinus tracts histologically showing a number of inter- connecting keratinized channels.

Papular scars are 3–4 mm skin-colored cobblestone-like papules. They are most commonly seen over nose, back, chin and mandibles.

Solid Facial Oedema (Morbihan Disease)[8]

This is a rare and disfiguring complication of acne that has been reported in twins. It is also reported as a consequence of rosacea and in Melkersson–Rosenthal syndrome. Thickened woody facial oedema leads to significant distortion of the midline face and cheeks due to soft-tissue swelling most likely due to pre-existing hypoplastic lymphatics. The disorder is frequently progressive, and the associated acne must be treated aggressively to prevent permanent swelling. Successful treatment with oral isotretinoin alone or in combination with clofazimine or ketotifen has been reported. Short or intermittent courses of oral steroids may also help the inflammatory component.

GRADES OF ACNE SCARRING

Goodman et al. proposed a qualitative grading system that differentiates four grades according to scar severity (Table 14.1). It is a simple grading system. Grade I corresponds to macular involvement (including erythematous, hyperpigmented or hypopigmented scars), whereas grades II, III, and IV correspond to mild, moderate and severe atrophic and hypertrophic lesions, respectively.[9] Interestingly, the authors consider severity of lesions according to visibility at a social distance (>50 cm).

Table 14.1: Goodman's qualitative global scarring grading system

Grade	*Level of disease*	*Characteristics*
1.	Macular disease	Erythematous, hyper- or hypopigmented flat marks visible to patient or observer at any distance.
2.	Mild disease	Mild atrophy or hypertrophy that may not be obvious at social distances of 50 cm or greater and may be covered adequately by makeup or the normal shadow of shaved beard hair in men or normal body hair if extra-facial.
3.	Moderate disease	Moderate atrophic or hypertrophic scarring that is obvious at social distances of 50 cm or greater and is not covered easily by makeup or the normal shadow of shaved beard hair in men or body hair if extra-facial, but is still able to be flattened by manual stretching of the skin (if atrophic).
4.	Severe disease	Severe atrophic or hypertrophic scarring that is obvious at social distances greater than 50 cm and is not covered easily by makeup or the normal shadow of shaved beard hair in men or body hair if extra-facial and is not able to be flattened by manual stretching of the skin.

Moreover, since patients may present with various types of acne scars at numerous anatomic sites (i.e. one cheek, the neck, the chest, and so on; these single areas are defined by the authors as "cosmetic units"). Scars are further subdivided into four grades of severity by anatomic sites involved, and the localized disease (up to three involved areas) is classified as A (1 cosmetic unit involvement) or B (2–3 cosmetic units), whereas the involvement of more cosmetic units is classified as generalized disease.

Authors also suggested a quantitative numeric grading system based on lesion counting (1–10, 11–20, >20), scar type (atrophic, macular, boxcar, hypertrophic, keloidal) and severity (mild, moderate and severe) (Table 14.2). Final scoring depends on the addition of points assigned to each respective category and reflects the disease severity ranging from minimum of 0 to maximum of 84.

Table 14.2: Goodman's quantitative global scarring grading system

Grade	*Type*	*Number of lesions 1(1–10)*	*Number of lesions 2 (11–20)*	*Number of lesions 3 (>20)*
1.	Milder scarring (1 point each) Macular erythematous pigmented Mildly atrophic dish-like	1 point	2 points	3 points
2.	Moderate scarring (2 points each) Moderately atrophic, dish like Punched out with shallow bases small scars (<5 mm) Shallow but broad atrophic areas	2 points	4 points	6 points
3.	Severe scarring (3 points each) Punched out with deep but normal bases, small scars (<5 mm) Punched out with deep but abnormal bases, small scars (<5 mm) Linear or troughed dermal scarring Deep, broad atrophic areas	3 points	6 points	9 points
4.	Hyperplastic Papular scars Keloidal/hypertrophic scars	2 points Area <5 mm^2 6 points	4 points Area 5–20 cm^2 12 points	6 points Area >20 cm^2 18 points

Dreno, et al. first proposed the ECLA scale (echelled' evaluation clinique des lesions d'acne), followed by the ECCA grading scale (echelled' evaluation clinique des cicatrices d'acné). According to this scoring system, morphological aspects of lesions define the type of scars as: Atrophic scars (V-shaped, U-shaped and M-shaped), superficial elastolysis, hypertrophic inflammatory scars (<2 years since onset), and keloid-hypertrophic scars (>2 years since onset). Each scar type is associated with a quantitative score (0, 1, 2, 3 depending on the

Table 14.3: ECCA (Echelled' evaluation clinique des Cicatrices d'acné) grading scale

Description factor (a)	*Weighing score (b)*	*Semiquantitative (a × b)*	*Grading*
V-shaped atrophic scars, diameter <2 mm, and punctiform	15	0 = no scar 1 = few scars 2 = limited number of scars 3 = many scars	/_/
U-shaped atrophic scars, diameter of 2–4 mm, with sheer edges	20	0 = no scar 1 = few scars 2 = limited number of scars 3 = many scars	/_/
M-shaped atrophic scars, diameter > 4 mm, superficial and with irregular surface	25	0 = no scar 1 = few scars 2 = limited number of scars 3 = many scars	/_/
Superficial elastolysis	30	0 = no scar 1 = few scars 2 = limited number of scars 3 = many scars	/_/
Subgrading 1 Hypertrophic inflammatory scars, scar of less than 2 years of age	40	0 = no scar 1 = few scars 2 = limited number of scars 3 = many scars	/_/
Keloid scars and hypertrophic scars that are more than 2 years of age	50	0 = no scar 1 = few scars 2 = limited number of scars 3 = many scars	/_/
Subgrading 2 Global score (Subgrading 1 + 2)			/_/

(*Source:* Dreno B, Khammari A, Orain N, et al. ECCA grading scale: an original validated acne scar grading scale for clinical practice in dermatology. Dermatology. 2007;214:46–51.)

number of lesions) multiplied by a weighing factor that varies according to severity, evolution, and morphological aspect. The final global score is directly correlated with clinical severity and ranges from 0 to 540 depending on the type and number of acne scars.

To summarize, there is a lack of consensus in the literature regarding acne scar nomenclature and classification.

A major problem is represented by the pleomorphic appearance of scars that may cause variable interpretation at clinical examination. A standard method for evaluation of scar depth represents an unmet need and is essential for therapeutic and prognostic purposes.

Ultrasound examination provides simple and reproducible quantitative parameters, representing a promising tool for a more accurate evaluation and classification of acne scars.

3-dimensional grid based mapping of lesions and moulded skin replicas have been devised for comparison.

Clinical Significance of Acne Scarring

Acne vulgaris is common condition of adolescence and early adulthood and scarring occurs in 95% of patients with acne, which is related to the time delay in seeking treatment.[9–11]

The physical blemish caused by the unsightly acne scar may be cosmetically, psychologically and socially disturbing to the patient.[12]

The negative psychosocial implications of acne are well documented and include association with both currently visible acne and sequel such as scarring.

Adverse psychosocial effects of acne that have been reported are social embarrassment, poor self-esteem, emotional debilitation, social isolation, avoidance of interpersonal interaction, diminished academic performance, altered perception of body image, anger, frustration, anxiety, depression and suicidal ideation.

Acne scarring represents the form of permanent sequelae from acne that is overall the most challenging to treat, as outcomes may be variable, and the extent of improvement is usually only partial, depending on the type and extent of scarring that is present.

No scar can ever be made to vanish completely; it can only be modified to make it cosmetically more aesthetic and functionally viable. Proper scar analysis should be made, object to be achieved should be outlined and all the available invasive and non-invasive modalities should be discussed with the patient before deciding the mode of correction.

Acne scar revision must basically improve the appearance without disturbing function. Its management must begin at the time of injury. Initial treatment, selection of the patient, timing of repair and proper technique are the important steps in its management.

REFERENCES

1. Farrar MD, Ingham E. Acne: inflammation. Clin Dermatol. 2004 Sep-Oct;22(5):380-4. doi: 10.1016/j.clindermatol.2004.03.006. PMID: 15556722.
2. Webster GF, Leyden JJ, Nilsson UR. Complement activation in acne vulgaris: consumption of complement by comedones. Infect Immun. 1979 Oct;26(1):183-6. doi: 10.1128/iai.26.1.183-186.1979. PMID: 159261; PMCID: PMC414592.
3. Jacob CI, Dover JS, Kaminer MS. Acne scarring: a classification system and review of treatment options. J Am Acad Dermatol. 2001 Jul;45(1):109-17. doi: 10.1067/mjd.2001.113451. PMID: 11423843.
4. Baum CL, Arpey CJ. Normal cutaneous wound healing: clinical correlation with cellular and molecular events. Dermatol Surg. 2005 Jun;31(6):674-86; discussion 686. doi: 10.1111/j.1524-4725.2005.31612. PMID: 15996419.
5. Kang S, Cho S, Chung JH, Hammerberg C, Fisher GJ, Voorhees JJ. Inflammation and extracellular matrix degradation mediated by activated transcription factors nuclear factor-kappaB and activator protein-1 in inflammatory acne lesions in vivo. Am J Pathol. 2005 Jun;166(6):1691-9. doi: 10.1016/s0002-9440(10)62479-0. PMID: 15920154; PMCID: PMC1602424.
6. Holland DB, Jeremy AH, Roberts SG, Seukeran DC, Layton AM, Cunliffe WJ. Inflammation in acne scarring: a comparison of the responses in lesions from patients prone and not prone to scar. Br J Dermatol. 2004 Jan;150(1):72-81. doi: 10.1111/j.1365-2133.2004.05749.x. PMID:14746619.
7. Rook's Textbook of dermatology–9th edition.
8. Donthi D, Nenow J, Samia A, Phillips C, Papalas J, Prenshaw K. Morbihan disease: a diagnostic dilemma: two cases with successful resolution. SAGE Open Medical Case Reports. 2021 Jun;9:2050313X211023655.

9. Goodman GJ, Baron JA. Postacne scarring: a qualitative global scarring grading system. Dermatol Surg. 2006 Dec;32(12):1458-66. doi: 10.1111/j.1524-4725.2006.32354.x. PMID: 17199653.
10. Prevalence, morbidity, and cost of dermatological diseases. J Invest Dermatol. 1979 Nov;73(5 Pt 2):395-401. doi: 10.1111/1523-1747.ep12541101. PMID: 501137.
11. Goulden V, Stables GI, Cunliffe WJ. Prevalence of facial acne in adults. J Am Acad Dermatol. 1999 Oct;41(4):577-80. PMID: 10495379.
12. Niemeier V, Kupfer J, Demmelbauer-Ebner M, Stangier U, Effendy I, Gieler U. Coping with acne vulgaris: evaluation of the chronic skin disorder questionnaire in patients with acne. Dermatology. 1998 Mar 13;196(1):108–15.

CHAPTER

15

Management of Acne Scar

INTRODUCTION

Post acne scarring is a very distressing and difficult problem for both physician and patients. Numerous invasive, semi-invasive and noninvasive techniques have been used to remove or replace acne scars, and in turn resurface the cutaneous surface and reduce shadows (Table 15.1).

Table 15.1: Effectivity of various treatment modalities in treatment of acne scars.[3]

Types of treatment	*Modality*[a]	*Ice-pick scars*	*Rolling scars*	*Shallow boxcar scars*	*Deep boxcar scars*
Resurfacing	Microdermabrasion				
	Dermabrasion				
	Peels				
	CROSS				
	Needling				
	Ablative laser				
Lifting-related	Subcision				
Volume-related	Filler				
	Platelet rich plasma[b]				
Skin tightening	Fractional/ nonablative lasers				

(Contd.)

Table 15.1: Effectivity of various treatment modalities in treatment of acne scars.[3] (*Contd.*)

Type of treatment	*Modality*[a]	*Ice-pick scars*	*Rolling scars*	*Shallow boxcar scars*	*Deep boxcar scars*
	Fractional radiofrequency	Less effective	Effective	Effective	Less effective
Surgery/ movement-related	Punch elevation	Ineffective	Ineffective	Effective	Effective
	Punch excision	Effective	Ineffective	Less effective	Effective

Effective | Less effective | Ineffective

CROSS: Chemical reconstruction of skin scars.

[a]Modalities with substantial quality of evidence data are included.

[b]Used as adjunct to other procedure.

The currently available treatments for acne scarring includes:[1, 2]

- **Aesthetic approach:** Chemical peels, microdermabrasion, dermal fillers, cryoslush.
- **Surgical approach:** Punch techniques, subcision, dermal grafting, fat transfer, implantation of autologous collagen, cultured and expanded autologous fibroblasts, microneedling, dermabrasion, scar revision.
- **Laser resurfacing** including ablative, non-ablative and fractional resurfacing.

CHEMICAL PEEL

Chemical peels are controlled chemical burns that are being increasingly used for acne, acne scar, hyperpigmentation and scars due to acne require medium depth peels.

AGENTS

Common agents used for chemical peels are Table 15.2:

- Glycolic acid (25–35%) (Fig. 15.1)
- Trichloroacetic acid (10%, 15%, 25%)
- Salicylic acid (20–30%)
- Jessner's peel

Table 15.2: Various peeling agents and depth of peel achieved				
Depth of peel	*Histological depth*	*GA*	*TCA*	*SA*
Very superficial	Stratum corneum	20–35%	10–15%	10–20%
Superficial	Epidermis	50–70%	15–20%	20–30%
Medium	Papillary dermis	70%	35–50%	30–50%

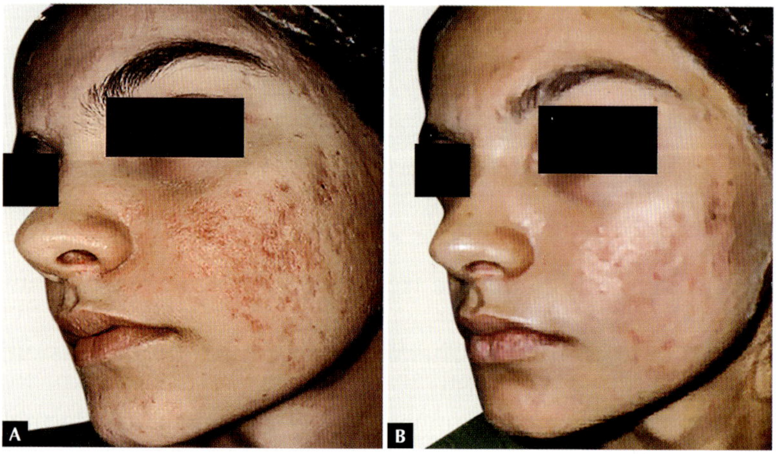

Fig. 15.1: Glycolic acid peel (35%): (A) At baseline; (B) After 6 sessions

Indication

Superficial and pigmented acne scars.

Mechanism of Action

1. Superficial peels cause exfoliation by keratolysis or decreased cellular adhesion.
2. Medium peels promote epidermal regeneration and collagen remodeling in papillary and upper reticular dermis and enhance glycosaminoglycans synthesis.
3. Deep peels cause deep reticular dermal regeneration.

Contraindications

- Active infection or wound
- Keloidal tendency
- Patient with unrealistic expectations

Side Effects

- Local irritation, burning, and pain
- Reactivation of herpes infection
- Persistent erythema
- Dyspigmentation
- Milia

MICRODERMABRASION

It has now lost the favor of being useful technique to address the acne scars.

Indications

Mainly used for the treatment of superficial acne scars and is ineffective for deeper scars.

The patient must be adequately counselled regarding the limitations of the procedure, the need for multiple sittings, and expected outcome and complications. The key to effective microdermabrasion is stretching the skin under tension for effective abrasion and achieving a vacuum to aspirate the epidermal debris and used crystals. Treatment is repeated weekly until the desired result is obtained.

Advantage

It is a safe procedure particularly in darker skin and requires no downtime.

Dermabrasion[3]

It has been used for several decades with good results however dermabrasion has been largely replaced by fractional lasers in the treatment of acne scarring.

Mechanism of Action

Removes the epidermis with or without part of the dermis, and the subsequent wound remodeling results in neocollagenesis, increased dermal thickness, and enhanced hydration and epidermal barrier.

Indications

- Well defined superficial scars with distinct borders.
- Broad based scars with indistinct borders.

Side effects

- Pain
- Erythema
- Dyspigmentation
- Significant recovery time
- Scarring from the procedure

MICRONEEDLING

The dermaroller is a hand held device with drum-shaped roller studded with 192 fine microneedles of 0.1 mm diameter in eight rows. The device is available in needle length ranging from 0.5 mm to 2 mm. Dermaroller with 1.5 mm needle length is commonly used in acne scar therapy (Fig. 15.2). Deeper atrophic scar may require 2 mm instrument. There are also motorized dermastamps and home care dermastamps available for percutaneous collagen induction. Motorized dermastamps are needle cartridges attached to a motor device similar to a mesogun having a to and fro movement inducing pricks. The speed and depth of the needling can be adjusted according to the scars.

Mechanism of action

- The upregulation of TGF-B3 through this process is thought to be the reason for natural collagen regeneration following needling

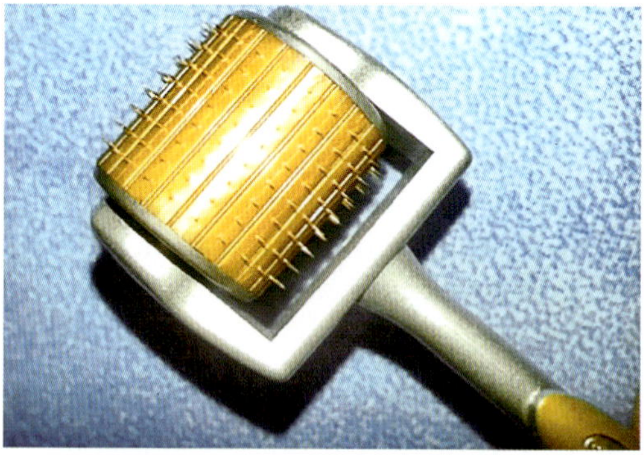

Fig. 15.2: Dermaroller instrument

- According to a newer theory, when microneedles penetrate the skin, they cause new wounds. Cells react to this intrusion with a "demarcation current" that is additionally increased by the needles' own electrical potential. This demarcation current (also called bioelectricity) triggers a cascade of growth factors that stimulate the healing phase.[4]

Indication

It is used for the rolling acne scars and box scars.

Procedure

The procedure is done under topical anesthesia. The facial skin is disinfected and anesthetized using a thick application of topical anesthetic cream. This is left for 30–45 minutes. The treatment is then carried out by rolling the needling tool over the areas affected by acne scars, four times in four different directions: Horizontally, vertically, and diagonally right and left. This ensures an even pricking pattern, resulting in about 250–300 pricks/cm^2. It has been shown that rolling with a dermaroller (192 needles, 200 mm length and 70 mm diameter) over an area for 15 times will result in approximately 250 holes/cm^2. The microneedles penetrate through the epidermis but do not remove it; the epidermis is only punctured and heals rapidly. As the needles are set in a roller, every needle initially penetrates at an angle and then goes deeper as the roller turns. Finally, the needle is extracted at a converse angle, therefore, curving the tracts and reflecting the path of the needle as it rolls into and then out of the skin for about 1.5–2 mm into the dermis. The epidermis, and particularly the stratum corneum, remains intact except for the minute holes, which are about four cells in diameter. Endpoint for each treatment is the presence of uniform bleeding points over the treated area (Fig. 15.3).

Contraindications

- Bleeding disorders
- Active herpes labialis

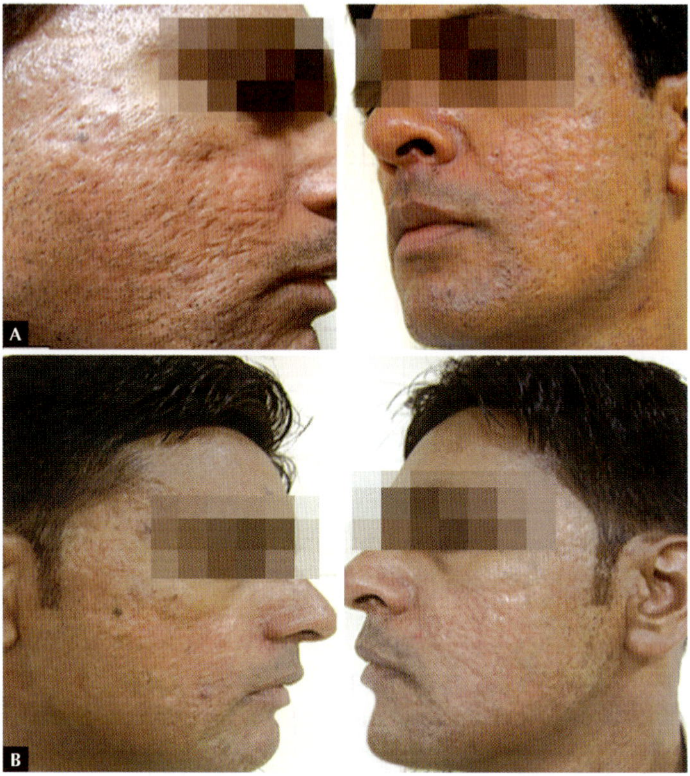

Fig. 15.3: Effect of dermaroller on acne scar: (A) Baseline; (B) After 5th sitting

- Patients on isotretinoin therapy
- Keloidal tendency

SUBCISION

Subcision also known as subcutaneous incisionless surgery is a surgical intervention used for the treatment of a variety of acne scars including atrophic scars and depressed scars.

Indications[4]

- Pitted acne scars before taking up for other procedures.
- Rolling acne scars-particularly scars that improve with stretching the skin.

Mechanism of Action

- Releasing fibrotic strands underlying scars.
- Organization of blood in the induced dermal pocket.
- Connective tissue formation in the area.

Needles which can be used in subcision are:

- Taylor's liberator (Fig. 15.4)
- Nokor needle (Fig. 15.5)
- 16–23 gauge needle

Procedure

Nokor needle is used. Needles ranging from 16 gauge to 23 gauge can be used in absence of Nokor needle. After topical anesthesia, the needle is inserted with blade facing upward, at the periphery of the scarred area. Afterwards, it is turned so that the tip is in a horizontal orientation just below dermal subcutaneous junction plane and gently swept across the site. A snapping sound is heard as the bands are broken. In addition, a gentle piston like (to and fro) motion has been used to advance needle through fibrous bands to release them. Firm pressure should be applied postoperatively for at least 5 minutes to achieve hemostasis. Treatment can be repeated at an interval of

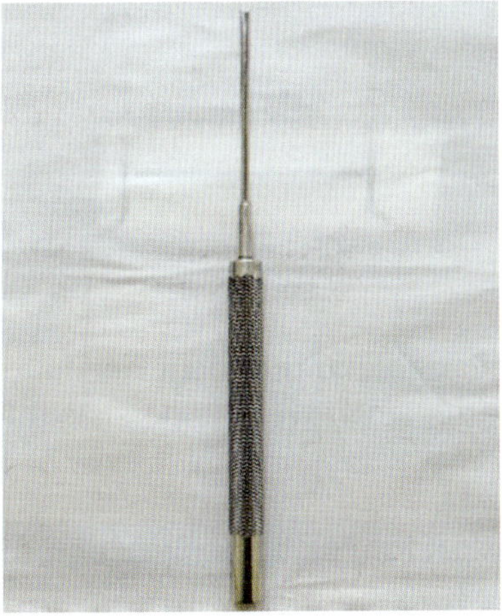

Fig. 15.4: Taylor's liberator

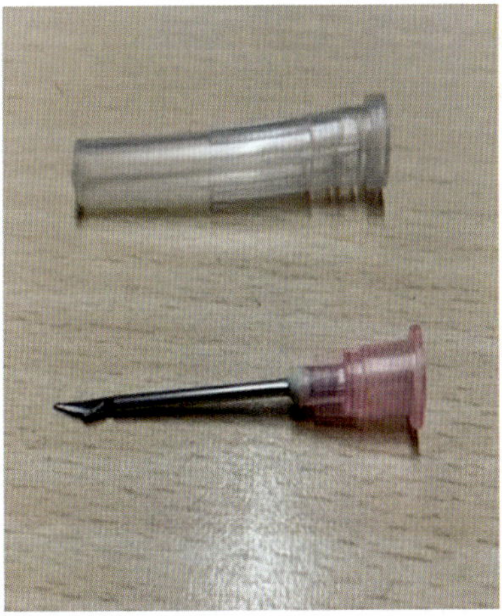

Fig. 15.5: Nokor neddle

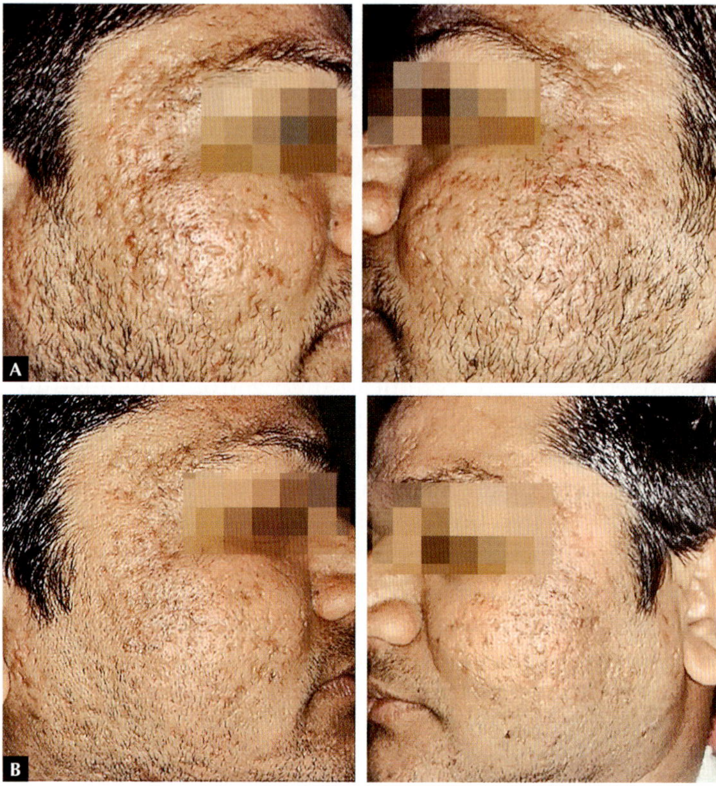

Fig. 15.6: Pre- and post-subcision pictures

6 weeks for up to two to three successive treatments (Figs 15.6 to 15.8).

Complications

- Bleeding and hematoma
- Some degree of swelling is invariable and patient needs to be counselled. Bluish discoloration and swelling persists for 5–7 days.

Radiofrequency-assisted Subcision for Postacne Scars

Here we make use of radiofrequency energy in place of mechanical energy for subcision.[5]

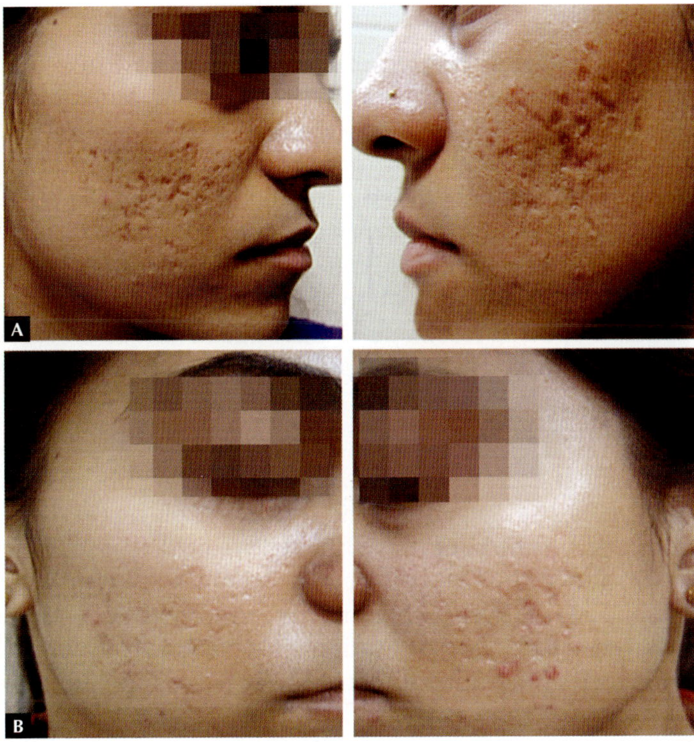

Fig. 15.7: Effect of subcision on acne scar: (A) Baseline; (B) After 4th sitting

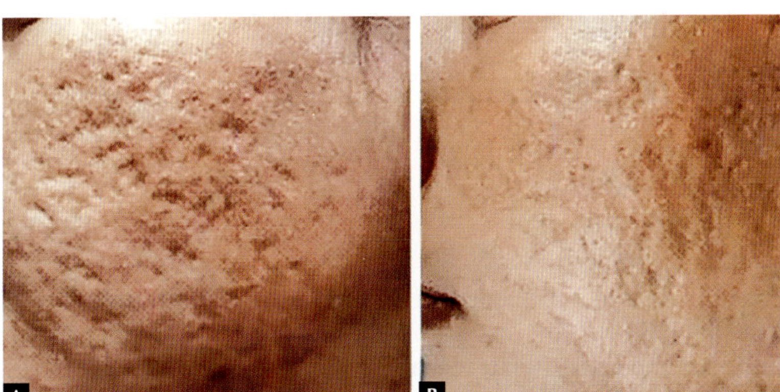

Fig. 15.8: Effect of dermaroller combined with subcision in acne scar (A) Sitting 1; (B) Sitting[4]

Procedure

A small window is created at the proximal end of a plastic sheath of an intravenous cannula. The intravenous cannula is introduced superficially into the scarred area parallel to the skin surface. The electrosurgery probe (in cutting mode, low power setting) is touched to the trochar of the cannula through the window. The fibrotic strands get cut with ease without any mechanical force as required in conventional subcision.[5]

RF subcision is a modification of above mentioned procedure, in which a special electrode is introduced under a scar and radiofrequency energy is passed through.

Mechanism of Action

The radiofrequency waves break the underlying fibrous tissue, thereby releasing and lifting the depressed scar, restoring the smooth contour of your skin. Blood vessels disrupted during the subcision allow blood to accumulate into the treated area. This blood clot prevents short-term reattachment of scars and contains growth factors for healing. This creates an environment for collagen regeneration and improving scar appearance over time.

The radiofrequency waves will also stimulate new collagen formations, improving; scars, skin complexion, lift & tighten skin, facial contouring, reducing wrinkles.

PUNCH TECHNIQUE

Types

- Punch excision
- Punch floatation
- Punch grafting

All punch techniques remove a pitted scar with a small rim of normal tissue. There are some scars, which are small, circular and punched out in appearance and have normal or altered texture of skin, like acne scars with white atrophic bases or sharply punched out "ice-pick" scars. Punch techniques can be used in the management of these scars.

Punch Excision

Indications

- Ice pick scar
- Deep boxcar scars less than 3.5 mm diameter

Procedure

After local anesthesia, scars are excised with a 1.5, 2, 2.5 or 3 mm biopsy punch as per size of the scar. By placing outward traction on the punch site at the time of excision, the circular wound is changed into an ellipse. To ensure that the ellipse runs parallel to the relaxed skin tension lines, the outward traction should be applied perpendicular to the skin lines. The scar tissue is removed and the wound sutured with one to three interrupted sutures using 6–0 nylon or prolene. If the punch excision is 2.5 mm or greater, a 6–0 vicryl (ethicon) subcutaneous suture can be placed prior to epidermal closure. This absorbable deep suture helps to promote wound edge eversion and facilitates proper healing.

Punch Floatation

Indication

Wide (>3 mm) boxcar acne scars that do not have significant color or texture.

Procedure

A punch size is selected to match the inner diameter of the crateriform scar. Now the punch is performed using a quick, rotating motion. It releases the bound-down scar. The plug is elevated with forceps and carefully freed from the underlying tissue. The plug is then elevated and positioned to lie slightly higher than the surrounding skin. The elevated punch can be secured in position by cyanoacrylate gel and closing with wound closure tapes like Steri-Strips.

Punch Grafting

Indication

Deep, irregular pits and tethered boxcar scars with altered skin texture.

Procedure

This is similar to that of the punch floatation, but replaces the plug with a donor plug instead of elevating the original defect. The scar plug is removed and a graft plug tissue is taken from the postauricular area or inner arm and grafted to the plug site. The donor punch graft should be 0.5 mm larger than the punch used to excise the scar. Graft is secured into place by cyanoacrylate tissue adhesive and wound closure tapes.

Limitation of Punch Techniques

- Punch replacement and punch flotation techniques are more successful for scars located on less mobile regions of the face such as the malar area and the forehead and less successful in perioral sites.
- Complications that may be observed include poor graft uptake, graft extrusion, and graft visibility. Poor color and textural mismatch are also frequently observed.
- Multiple procedures may be needed.
- Recently with the availability of lasers, these procedures are performed less frequently.

CHEMICAL RECONSTRUCTION OF SKIN SCARS

Chemical reconstruction of skin scars (CROSS) is a technique using high strength TCA focally on the atrophic acne scars. Trichloroacetic acid is a versatile peeling agent because the peel depth varies according to its concentration. It is also self-neutralizing and not absorbed in the systemic circulation; hence, high concentrations can be safely used without risk of systemic absorption.

Mechanism of Action

Application of the caustic agent TCA causes precipitation of proteins, coagulative necrosis of cells in the epidermis, and necrosis of collagen in the papillary to upper reticular dermis.[6] There is an increase in dermal volume as a result of an increase in collagen production, glycosaminoglycans, elastin fragmentation and reorganization of dermal collagen. The dermal remodeling continues for several months. During the remodeling phase, type III collagen is gradually replaced by type I collagen. The fibroblasts are oriented parallel to the epidermis which leads to improvement of scars.

Indication

Ice-pick scars.

Procedure

The scars are marked with a surgical marking pen. The face is cleaned with spirit and degreased with acetone. The procedure is carried out with the patient sitting comfortably as lying down can cause effacement of appearance of the scars. The skin is stretched, and 100% TCA is focally applied with a wooden toothpick pressing firmly up to the bottom of the depressed scar taking care to avoid spillage to the surrounding skin. Nowadays 20% and 50% TCA is also used. The skin is monitored carefully and kept stretched until a frosted appearance is seen. Frosting is a result of coagulation of epidermal and dermal proteins and is generally seen in 10–15 seconds. The patient is asked to wash the face after the procedure. Photoprotection is recommended. TCA CROSS can be repeated at 4 weeks interval for a total of three treatments.

Complications

Transient postinflammatory hyperpigmentation and hypopigmentation even depigmentation.

DERMAL FILLERS

A dermal filler is a natural or synthetic collagen used for injection in the dermis for the augmentation of soft tissue. Dermal fillers are now frequently used for acne scars.

Fillers containing hyaluronic acid, calcium hydroxyapatite, and poly-L-lactic acid (PLLA) are increasingly used to correct atrophic acne scarring. Injection of cross-linked hyaluronic acid enhances collagen formation by dermal fibroblasts and improves the quality of overlying skin.[3]

An ideal dermal filler should be safe, effective, non-carcinogenic, non-teratogenic, inert and durable. Dermal filler can be classified based on:

- Origin (natural/synthetic).
- Source (autograft/allograft/heterograft).
- Content (collagen/fat/hyaluronic acid/silicon/peptides).
- Duration of effect (temporary/permanent).

Procedure

The injection technique is the standard method of dermal fillers. The implant material available in the prefilled syringe, is injected in the superficial dermis with a 32 G needle. It permits free flow of the implant material in the upper dermis to correct soft tissue defect. If required, material can also be uniformly spread by very gentle manipulation.

Adverse Effects

- Bruising
- Secondary bacterial infection.
- Cyst and abscess formation.
- Reactivation of herpes infection.
- Local tissue necrosis due to vascular occlusion.
- Blindness due to retinal artery embolism.

BIOFILLERS

Biofiller gel is autologous and easy to obtain. The consistency and autologous nature of plasma biofiller are better accepted by patients than the high density hyaluronic acid fillers.[7]

Procedure

- Topical 2.5% lidocaine plus 2.5% prilocaine anesthetic cream was applied over the patient's face.
- 10 ml of patient's blood was drawn and mixed with 1 ml anticoagulant acid citrate dextrose. It was rotated at 3200 rotations per minute (RPM) for 8 min in a centrifuge machine. The plasma solution was withdrawn and centrifuged again at 1000 RPM for 5 min. The upper part that is platelet-poor plasma (PPP) was withdrawn in a 5 ml syringe, approximately 4.5 ml, and the lower part that is PRP was withdrawn in 3 insulin (1 ml) syringes, approximately 2.5 ml.

- Calcium gluconate was added in the PPP in the proportion of 0.01 ml/1 ml of PPP. It was incubated in hot water (heated in a metal container) at 100°C (gradually reducing to 98°C) for 5 min and then in cold water bath in a metal container with initial temperature 7°C and gradually increasing to 10°C for 5 min.
- The viscous gel, approximately 3 ml in volume, will be formed as shown in Fig. 15.9.[7]

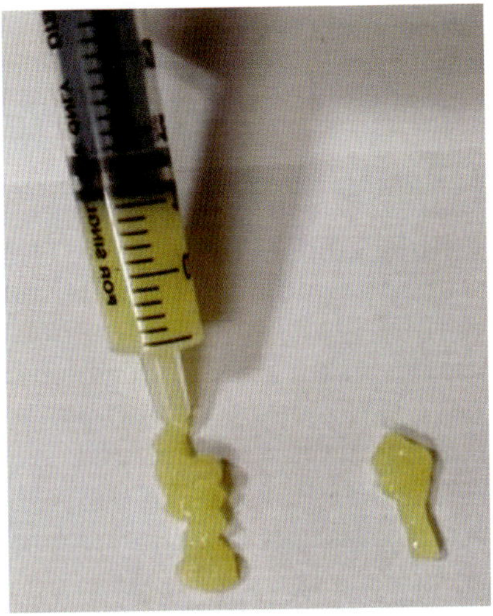

Fig. 15.9: Showing biofiller made from PPP (platelet poor plasma)[7]

Advantages of Biofillers[7]

- PPP gel injection as a dermal filler is a cost-effective, well-tolerated, very simple nonsurgical clinic procedure.
- It is an autologous material easily obtained from the patient's own blood, and therefore, any risks of immunogenic reactions or disease transmission are eliminated.

Disadvantages of Biofillers

- Complete response takes 3–6 months.
- Less effective.

AUTOLOGOUS FAT GRAFTING

Fat stores are abundant with adipose derived stem cells, which can generate epithelial hyperplasia and angiogenesis. Release of growth factors like VEGF, PDGF, TGF-b, MMP, IGF-1, BGFG and BDNF stimulate endothelial cells, fibroblasts and tissue progenitor cells to remodel scar tissue.[8]

AFG has the advantage of being easily available and can be injected in multiple sites of the body. Furthermore, it is not immunogenic, is easily available. The volume filling capabilities allow the natural contours of skin to be regained while counteracting the depressive and retracted nature of scar tissue.[8]

DERMAL GRAFTING

Dermal graft is effective as a filler material for treating depressed scars. It builds on previous subcision and consists of placing dermal grafts into precise pockets under the skin. A dermal graft is a skin graft from which epidermis and subcutaneous fat have been removed. Survival rates of dermal grafts are much higher than fat transplant.

Dermal grafting can be used to treat any round/oval facial scar that is soft, prominent, and at least 4–5 mm[3].

Advantages of Using Dermal Graft

- Readily available material
- Easy to perform
- Not susceptible to infection
- Can be accurately tailored for a variety of defects
- Creates a permanent spacer between overlying skin and underlying fibrous band of tissue.

Disadvantages of Using Dermal Graft[3]

- It involves multiple incisions that generate new scar.
- Occasional granuloma formation can occur secondary to transplantation of epidermis from the donor site into the recipient site.

Procedure

Types of Technique

- Conventional
- Enzymatic

Conventional Technique: Procedure

After local anesthesia, the scar is subcised using the 18 gauge or Nokor needle 10–14 days before the operation in order to stimulate granulation tissue and achieve some initial correction.

Donor tissue is harvested using any conventional dermatomes or using biopsy punches from the postauricular site down to the fascia level. The epidermal part is trimmed using fine scissors. Alternatively, dermal tissue can also be harvested from a dermabraded area where the whole of epidermis is completely removed. Excess of fat is also trimmed in the similar way. Derma-fat graft can be used in larger defects. These punches or long narrow strip of dermis are transferred to saline. The defective area is tunnelled to create a space for the graft; as per the size of the defect. A small slit is made to insert the grafts. The grafts are trimmed according to the shape of the defect. The graft is inserted using a forceps and once complete correction has occurred, the slit is sutured with proline.

Enzymatic Technique: Procedure

Here trypsin is used to make the firm dermal tissue soft and mouldable. Full thickness skin graft is harvested as in case of conventional technique. This is then transferred into a petridish containing 0.25% of trypsin in EDTA solution. This is incubated at 37°C for 75 minutes. After incubation, the tissue is transferred to phosphate buffered saline and the epidermis is manually separated. The dermal tissue separated by enzymatic technique is soft, flexible and easily mouldable in comparison with the firm dermal tissue harvested by the conventional technique. This is filled into the defect as in case of conventional technique. Or it can be transferred into 1cc syringe and pushed into the defect. Area can be moulded by external manipulation. The slit made for inserting the material is then sutured.

SCAR REVISION

In selected cases, when scarring is linear and extensive, scar revision techniques such as Z, M and Y plasty may be useful. These need to be performed by a dermatosurgeon properly trained in performing these procedures.

Cryotherapy

Indications

For papular and hypertrophic scars.

Cryoslush and cryopeel are used for the treatment of nodulocystic acne, inflammatory papule and pustule.

Cryoslush Method

Solid CO_2 is crushed and a few drops of acetone are added to make a paste. This paste is rapidly applied to the lesions with a gauze ball for 2–10 seconds. Superficial peeling is achieved due to epidermal necrosis, which causes desquamation of comedones, resolution of inflammatory papules, pustules, nodules and cysts.

Cryopeel Method

A spray of liquid nitrogen is used for 2–3 seconds, instead of CO_2 slush. However, pigmentary changes are commonly observed, particularly in darker-skinned patients and so this procedure should be used carefully only after proper counseling of the patient. Persistent erythema and scarring may also occur.

Platelet-Rich Plasma

It is helpful in boxcar and rolling scars but shows limited efficacy in ice-pick scars.

It can be effectively combined with needling for better outcomes.[3]

LASER TREATMENT

Indication

1. Scars causing a significant psychological impact.
2. Patients with Grade 2 and Grade 3 scars by the Goodman and Baron grading system.[9]
3. All patients with boxcar scars (superficial or deep) or rolling scars.[10]

Types of Laser

Ablative Lasers

Ablative lasers cause an injury or ablation of the epidermis and a part of the dermis with resultant collagen deposition. This collagen deposition in the dermis along with a renewal of the epidermal layer is responsible for amelioration of post-acne atrophic scars as well as any pigment dyschromias. Carbon dioxide laser and Erbium YAG (Er: YAG) laser are the most commonly used ablative lasers for the treatment of acne scars.

CO_2 lasers have a double effect—they promote the wound healing process and arouse an amplified production of myofibroblasts and matrix proteins such as hyaluronic acid (Fig. 15.10 A and B).

Patients with a Fitzpatrick skin types 4, 5 and 6 are prone to develop hyperpigmentation after treatment than patients with low phototype.

Complications of laser resurfacing are caused by:

- Too deep treatment
- Delivering higher energy
- Poor post resurfacing wound care
- Improper patient selection
- Poor patient compliance

Non-ablative Lasers

Non-ablative lasers induce controlled injury to the dermal collagen without any damage to the epidermis. This leads to a healing response with dermal collagen remodeling which causes a tightening effect on the skin with resultant improvement in the appearance of the scars.

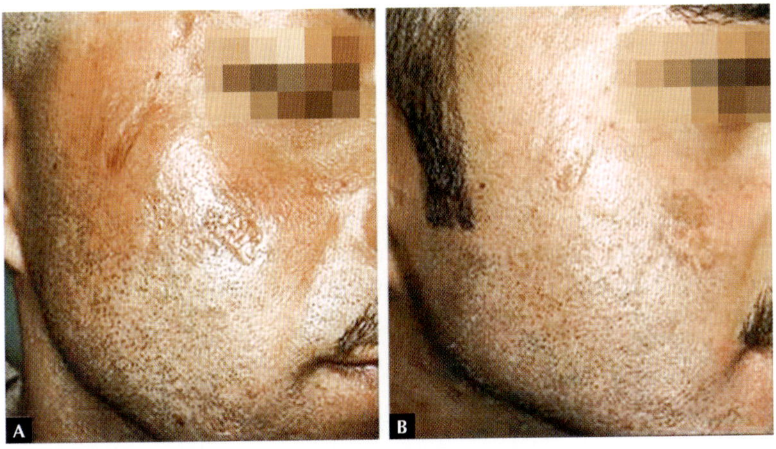

Fig. 15.10A and B: (A) Pre- and (B) post-ablative laser pictures

Non-ablative lasers for acne scars are of two types:

a. **Infrared lasers:** 1,450 nm diode laser, 1,064 nm Q-switched Nd: YAG laser, 1,320 nm Nd: YAG laser and 1,540 nm Er: glass laser.
b. **Visible light lasers:** Commonly used intense pulsed light (specially for hypertrophic scar and keloids), pulsed dye lasers, light emitting diodes, broadband light sources, etc.

Non-ablative lasers decrease the risk of side effects and the need for postoperative care but have limited efficacy.

Fractional Photothermolysis

Pigmentary abnormalities following laser treatment is always a cause of concern. Newer modalities using the principles of fractional photothermolysis (FP) devices to create patterns of tiny microscopic wounds surrounded by undamaged tissues are the devices that are now preferred for scar treatments. Unlike selective photothermolysis, which produces bulk thermal injury to specific targets in the skin, fractional photothermolysis (fraxel, reliant technologies, Inc., mountain view, CA) creates hundreds of microthermal treatment zones (MTZs) while sparing the surrounding tissue. FP creates microscopic thermal wounds and specifically spares tissue surrounding each wound. The microscopic treatment zones form the building blocks for a macroscopic treatment effect.

MTZs are intentionally made to be so small that they can barely be seen, if at all, without magnification. The macroscopic treatment effect of FP is characterized both by the arrangement and shape of these microscopic treatment zones within the skin. Laser parameters can be adjusted to produce different three-dimensional (3-D) MTZ shapes and depths. Thus, the skin can be treated primarily or "touched up" in a digital manner based on the density of the microscopic treatment zones.

Combination Therapy

All the procedures can be utilised in combination so as to achieve best therapeutic outcome.

- Subcision, the process by which there is separation of the acne scar from the underlying skin. Subcision releases the scars from the underlying adhesions which should be the first step for any treatment for acne scars.
- Peeling with trichloroacetic acid.
- Lastly, fractional laser irradiation.

The duration of combination therapy is variable for the given patient. Triple combination therapy is a safe and very effective combination treatment modality for a variety of atrophic acne scars.

HYPERTROPHIC SCARS

Silicone Gel

Silicone-based products represent one of the most common and effective solutions in preventing and also in the treatment of hypertrophic acne scars.

Advantages

It is transparent, quick drying, nonirritating and does not induce skin maceration, it can be used to treat extensive scars and uneven areas of skin.

Mechanism of Action

It is not fully understood but several hypotheses have been proposed:

1. Increase in hydration
2. Increase in temperature
3. Protection of the scar
4. Alter secretion of growth factors which further affects the fibrosis

Treatment with silicone gel can be used in patients of any age and women of childbearing age. Moreover, the silicone gel can be used throughout the year, including summer. It is costly therapy.

INTRALESIONAL STEROID THERAPY

Intralesional injection of steroids is one of the most common treatments for keloids and hypertrophic scars.

Mechanism of Action

- Corticosteroids may reduce the volume, thickness, and texture of scars, and they can relieve symptoms such as itching and discomfort.
- In addition to their anti-inflammatory properties, steroids exert a vasoconstrictor and an antimitotic activity.
- Steroids suppress inflammation by inhibition of leukocytes and monocyte migration, vasoconstriction and anti-mitotic effect, inhibit keratinocyte and fibroblast proliferation. They also reduce plasma protease inhibitors concentration so that collagenase degrades collagen.

Intralesional steroid therapy may be preceded by a light cryotherapy with liquid nitrogen, 10–15 minutes before injection, to improve the dispersion of the drug in scar tissue and minimize the deposition in the subcutaneous and perilesional tissue. The steroid that is currently most frequently used in the treatment of hypertrophic scars and keloid is triamcinolone acetonide (10–40 mg/ml).

Adverse Reactions

- Hypopigmentation
- Skin atrophy
- Pain
- Telangiectasia
- Infections

Cryotherapy

For hypertrophic scars and keloids, the low temperature reached during cryotherapy sessions cause a slowing of blood flow and cause the formation of intraluminal thrombus leading to anoxia and tissue necrosis. Younger and smaller scars are most responsive to cryotherapy.

Cryotherapy is significantly more effective than alternative methods for richly vascularized keloids. During each session of cryotherapy the patient is usually subjected to 2–3 cycles, each lasting less than 5–30 seconds.

For the localized lesions on the face, freezing and pain restrict the use of cryotherapy in these areas, especially in cases where the scars are numerous.

Therefore, cryotherapy can be taken into consideration especially for scars located on the trunk or for particularly bulky scars on the face.

Complications

- Hypo- and hyperpigmentation
- Skin atrophy
- Pain

Papular Acne Scars

Papular acne scars are skin-colored, minimally raised, 3–4 mm discrete, cobblestone-like papules most commonly present on back, nose, and chin Fig. 15.11.

Normal radiofrequency (RF) ablation of even superficial lesions such as papular acne scars can lead to scarring and pigmentation. Intralesional RF (ILRF) targets only the deeper reticular dermis, thus minimizing the scarring of the epidermal tissue.[11]

Procedure

A small window is created at the proximal end of plastic sheath of intravenous (IV) cannula (22G, blue). The tip of cannula is inserted into the center of the papule. Depth of the tip depends on the size of lesion. Electric current is passed from RF probe to IV cannula by touching the tip of probe to the cannula through the window created.

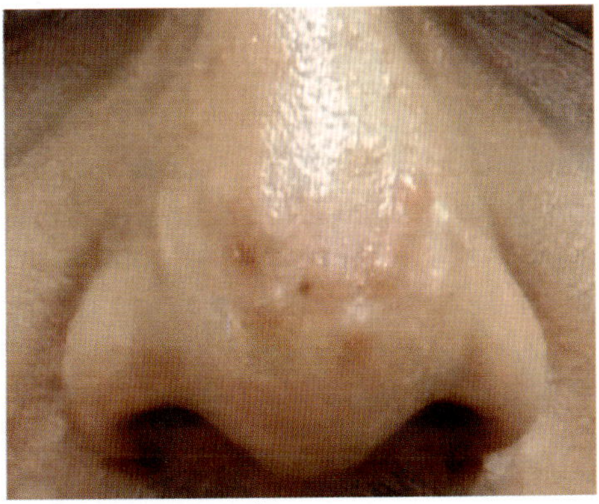

Fig. 15.11: Papular acne scar over nose

ILRF targets only the deeper reticular dermis, thus minimizing the scarring of the epidermal tissue.[11]

Pinhole Method Using an Erbium: YAG Laser for the Treatment of Papular Acne Scars

The pinhole method using an Er:YAG laser creates multiple tiny holes that penetrate from the epidermis into the deeper dermis. The 2,940 nm Er:YAG laser is well suited for skin resurfacing due to its high water affinity The pinhole method using an Er:YAG laser improves the scar height and texture by inducing collagen bundle regeneration and realignment following the physical breakage and thermal damage. The main benefit of this method includes the ability to adjust the small holes for individual scar types.[12]

Ablative Carbon Dioxide Laser Treatment for Papular Acne Scars

Ablative carbon dioxide laser therapy (10,600 nm, continuous mode, energy of 15 W) was performed under topical anesthesia. The lesions were ablated until they completely disappeared. After laser treatment, the lesions healed with buildup of some scar tissue, but not to the original severity. Chances of post-laser hyperpigmentation, hypopigmentation, or infection is rare.[13]

THREAD LIFTING

Thread lifting is a simple non-surgical facelift procedure in which a long barbed suture is inserted through the face and into the subcutaneous layer.

It not only mechanically lifts the skin but also triggers collagen synthesis through fibroblast activation.

Originally, this was achieved with nonabsorbable threads, whose resistance to biodegradation and high tensile strength provide long-term cosmetic improvement.

Despite their high duration of clinical efficacy, however, nonabsorbable threads have largely been replaced by less permanent absorbable threads, which yield shorter-term correction but offer greater biocompatibility and lower risk of infection.[14]

BOTULINUM TOXIN[3]

As severely atrophic (grade 3) acne scars can be aggravated by normal muscle movement, several authors find that botulinum toxin can be beneficial, especially for acne scars in areas such as the forehead, glabella, and chin.

NOVEL MODALITIES[3]

Autologous bone marrow stem cell intradermal injection has been found to be safe and effective for all types of atrophic scars. Intradermal autologous fibroblast injections are a well tolerated treatment option for depressed distensible acne scars.

Topical epidermal growth factor (EGF) was recently used to improve atrophic acne scars in patients.

EXOSOMES

Exosomes are cell-derived nanoscale vesicles carrying various biomolecules, including proteins, nucleic acids, and lipids, with the capability to communicate with adjacent or distant cells.[15]

Applications of human adipose tissue stem cell-derived exosomes have been suggested as novel cell-free therapeutic strategies in acne scar. Combined use of this novel material with resurfacing devices like fractional CO_2 or microneedling would provide synergistic effects on both the efficacy and safety of atrophic acne scar treatments.[16]

REFERENCES

1. Jacob CI, Dover JS, Kaminer MS. Acne scarring. A classification system and review of treatment options. J Am Acad Dermatol. 2001;45:109–17.
2. Alster TS. Cutaneous resurfacing with CO_2 and erbium: YAG lasers: Preoperative, intraoperative and postoperative considerations. Plast Reconstr Surg. 1999;103:619.
3. Bhargava S, Cunha PR, Lee J, Kroumpouzos G. Acne scarring management: systematic review and evaluation of the evidence. American Journal of Clinical Dermatology. 2018 Aug;19:459–77.
4. Liebl H. (2006). Abstract reections about collagen- induction therapy (CIT). A hypothesis for the mechanism of action of collagen induction therapy (CIT) using microneedles. Available from www.dermaroller.de/us/science/abstractreflections-26.html. [Accessed January, 2012].

5. Yadav S, Gupta S. Radiofrequency-assisted subcision for postacne scars. Journal of the American Academy of Dermatology. 2018 Jan 1;78(1):e9–10.
6. Yug A, Lane JE, Howard MS, et al. Histologic study of depressed acne scars treated with serial high-concentration (95%) trichloroacetic acid. Dermatol Surg. 2006;32: 985–90.
7. Gupta S, Bisht PB, Kannan C. Bio-filler: an effective facial rejuvenation tool—easy on pocket. Journal of Cutaneous and Aesthetic Surgery. 2020 Jul;13(3):243.
8. Riyat H, Touil LL, Briggs M, Shokrollahi K. Autologous fat grafting for scars, healing and pain: a review. Scars, burns & healing. 2017 Sep 14;3:2059513117728200.
9. Alster T, Zaulyanov L. Laser scar revision: a review. Dermatol Surg. 2007;33:131–40.
10. Khan MH, Sink RK, Manstein D, et al. Intradermally focused infrared laser pulses: thermal effects at defined tissue depths. Lasers Surg Med. 2005;36:270–80.
11. Sanke S, Chander R, Mehra S. Intralesional radiofrequency for papular acne scars. Indian Dermatology Online Journal. 2019 Jul;10(4):486.
12. Lee SJ, Kim JM, Kim YK, Seo SJ, Park KY. The pinhole method using an erbium: YAG laser for the treatment of papular acne scars. Dermatologic Therapy. 2017 Sep;30(5):e12512.
13. Fonseka S, Wickramaarachchi DC, Bandara DD. Ablative carbon dioxide laser treatment for papular scars of nose and chin due to acne: a case series. International Journal of Dermatology and Venereology. 2021 Sep 30;4(03):182–4.
14. Tam C, Khong J, Tam K, Vasilev R, Wu W, Hazany S. A comprehensive review of non-energy-based treatments for atrophic acne scarring. Clinical, Cosmetic and Investigational Dermatology. 2022 Mar 14:455–69.
15. Xiong M, Zhang Q, Hu W, Zhao C, Lv W, Yi Y, Wang Y, Tang H, Wu M, Wu Y. The novel mechanisms and applications of exosomes in dermatology and cutaneous medical aesthetics. Pharmacological research. 2021 Apr 1;166:105490.
16. Kwon HH, Yang SH, Lee J, Park BC, Park KY, Jung JY, Bae Y, Park GH. Combination treatment with human adipose tissue stem cell-derived exosomes and fractional CO_2 laser for acne scars: a 12-week prospective, double-blind, randomized, split-face study. Acta Dermato-Venereologica. 2020 Nov 4;100(18):1–8.

CHAPTER 16

Lasers and Light in Acne

Laser and light-based acne treatments are increasingly becoming first choice of laser physicians to treat acne as well as acne scars. It may be an alternative to medical treatment for nonresponders and is associated with minimal adverse effects if used judiciously. These devices also offer an option for those patients who have moderate to severe acne but are concerned about oral medications.

Long-term improvements have been documented with laser treatments. Compared with light therapy, lasers have the advantage to concentrate coherent light on a smaller area of tissue.

A variety of light and laser devices has been used for the treatment of acne, including the fractional CO_2 laser potassium titanyl phosphate (KTP) laser, the 585 nm and 595 nm pulsed dye lasers, the 1450 nm diode laser, radio-frequency devices, intense pulsed light sources, low-intensity light treatment, and photo-dynamic therapy using 5-aminolevulinic acid and indocya-nine green.

The various light sources include fluorescent, halogen, xenon, tungsten lamps, and recently lasers. The devices used to treat acne may be separated into groups based on approach.

Devices that directly or indirectly target in *P. acnes*:

- UVA-excites the porphyrins in *P. acnes*, killing it
- Blue light
- Blue and red light combination

Devices that alter the sebaceous gland structure:

- Aminolevulinic acid (ALA) and photodynamic therapy (PDT)

- Infrared lasers
- Radiofrequency

Devices that exert an effect on both:

- Pulse dye laser (PDL)
- Potassium titanyl phosphate (KTP) laser target
- Intense pulsed light (IPL).

FRACTIONAL CO_2 LASER

Among all ablative and non-ablative fractional lasers 1–3 the one that has been the most commonly used and reported successful is the fractional CO_2. A number of clinical studies have confirmed the efficacy of this laser system in acne scars.

Steps of Fractional Laser in Treatment of Acne Scars

- The procedure is done usually under the effect of topical anesthesia under occlusion. An eutectic mixture of prilocaine/tetracaine and lignocaine is commonly used and kept for 45 minutes to 1 hour.
- A proper fluence and density settings are then selected according to the scar type and severity.
- Deeper scars need higher fluencies as the depth of penetration of the laser beam is directly proportional to it. It is important to treat the shoulder or margins of scars to achieve a good therapeutic benefit.
- A topical non-comedogenic antibiotic cream is advised in the postoperative period. Patients are advised to avoid sun exposure after the procedure to minimize the chances of post-inflammatory hyperpigmentation.

532 nm POTASSIUM TITANYL PHOSPHATE LASER

The potassium titanyl phosphate (KTP) vascular laser has generally been used for the treatment of telangiectasis and rosacea but has also recently been shown to be effective for the treatment of acne. Although the exact mechanism of action is unclear, selective photothermolysis of blood vessels with deeper penetration than blue light and activation of porphyrins to target *P. acnes* and/or collateral thermal damage to sebaceous glands have all been postulated. KTP has been shown to have short-term effects on improving acne severity with minimal side effects.

585 nm and 595 nm PULSED DYE LASER

As with the KTP laser, the pulsed dye laser has been used mainly for the selective photothermolysis of vascular disorders, as well as other inflammatory disorders such as psoriasis and telangiectatic rosacea. In addition, the pulsed dye laser is widely known to stimulate dermal remodeling and collagen production. It has been used for the treatment of hypertrophic scar, keloids, as well as, **acne scarring**.

The effect of this laser on acne is believed to be mediated by decreasing *P. acnes* density or sebaceous gland activity. Its action targeting oxyhemoglobin has also been investigated for treatment of acne. It causes selective photothermolysis of the dilated vascular component of inflammation associated with acne. Through the delivery of coherent yellow light, porphyrins are activated to produce phototoxic effects.

Some studies suggest that, it leads to significant upregulation of transforming growth factor b, which is a potent stimulator of neocollagenesis and a potent inhibitor of inflammation.

1450 nm DIODE LASER

This device can cause thermal coagulation of the sebaceous lobule and associated hair follicle through peak thermal heating of the upper to mid dermis up to a depth of 500 μm. The presumed mechanism of acne improvement is through heating of the sebaceous gland and associated structures resulting in reduced sebaceous gland activity resulting in a reduction in inflammatory acne lesions.

Treatment with the infrared 1450 nm diode laser with a dynamic cooling device has been shown to safely and effectively reduce inflammatory acne lesions of the face with fluences as high as 14 $J/cm.^2$

1540 nm ERBIUM GLASS LASER

A single study has also shown efficacy of the 1540 nm erbium glass laser for treatment of acne. After four treatments at 4-week intervals, a 78% reduction in acne lesions and decreased skin oiliness was noted in 25 patients.

INTENSE PULSED LIGHT

Unlike a laser, an intense pulsed light source provide a non-coherent (500 to 1200 nm) source of intense light that can be modified by filters to provide irradiation with specific wavelengths of light. The use of intense pulsed light for the treatment of acne has been theoretically based on the production of singlet oxygen after photoactivation of porphyrins synthesized and stored by *P. acnes*.

Broad spectrum delivery by IPL devices is believed to lead to photothermolysis, where the absorption of light by endogenous chromophores in the skin creates enough heat and energy to target the blood vessels that supply sebaceous glands in order to reduce sebum production.

In comparison with other light sources, IPL was less effective at reducing acne lesions than pulsed dye lasers but more effective than blue-red combination light-emitting diodes.

Common adverse effects of IPL are pain, swelling, erythema, burn blistering and crusting.

A combined radiofrequency and pulsed light device has recently been used to treat acne. Reduction in perifollicular inflammation and sebaceous glands is the presumed mechanism of action. Side effects observed are erythema, tingling and burning.

TARGETING *P. ACNES*

P. acnes is implicated in the pathogenesis of acne. It is a Gram-positive micro-aerophilic skin bacterium. It is known to produce and accumulate endogenous porphyrins, namely protoporphyrin, uroporphyrin, and coproporphyrin III during its normal metabolism and reproduction. These porphyrins absorb light energy at the near-ultraviolet (UV) and blue light spectrum which induces these photosensitizers to generate highly reactive free radical species subsequently causing destruction of lipids in the cell wall of *P. acnes* and ultimately bacterial destruction. Although this process of absorption

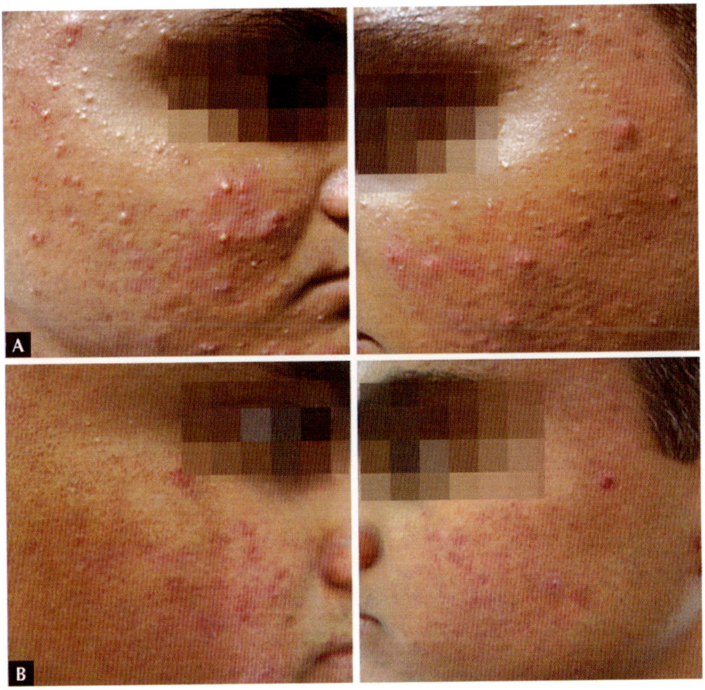

Fig. 16.1: Effect of IPL in acne: (A) Baseline; (B) After 6th sitting

and photodynamic excitation is highly efficient between the wavelengths of 400 and 430 nm, with enough light, the reaction may be induced with a variety of different wavelengths. Many light sources may affect *P. acnes* including KTP lasers (532 nm), PDLs (585–595 nm), narrowband light sources, IPL devices (broadband light) and various orange/red light lasers or light sources (610–635 nm).

MICRONEEDLE RADIOFREQUENCY (MNRF)[4]

Fractional MNRF device works by creating radiofrequency thermal zones without epidermal injury that ultimately lead to long-term and controlled dermal remodeling in the form of neoelastogenesis and neocollagenesis.

Needle tip contains tiny gold needles acting as an internal conductor. It gives a more uniform deep tissue warming that will stimulate collagen and new collagen fibres.

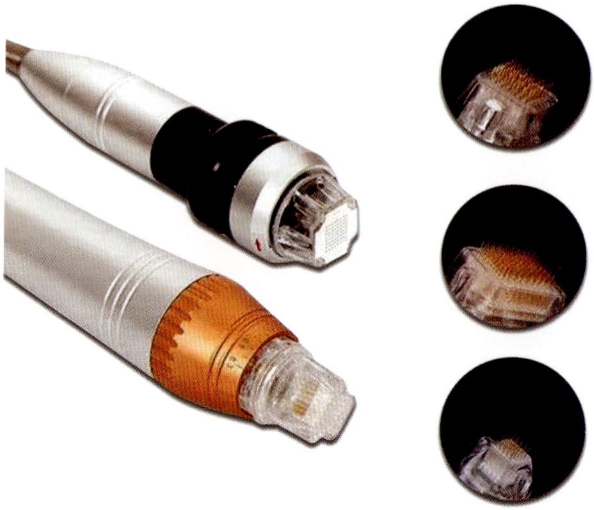

Fig. 16.2: Probes and needle used in microneedle radiofrequency

The electrical energy is transposed into thermal energy. As the needles are insulated apart from their tips, the micro- holes created are not exposed to thermal damage during the RF emission, which minimise the side effects of pigmentation spares any damage to epidermis.

UVA/UVB

An improvement in acne was reported in about 70% of patients after sunlight exposure, but it was unclear up to recently as to which wavelengths contributed to this favorable effect, UV, visible light, or the combination of both. UVA and UVB treatment showed a marginal beneficial effect, but it is potentially carcinogenic.

Blue Light and Red Light

Blue light has the most effective visible wavelength for photoactivation of endogenous porphyrin component of *P. acnes* because the 407 nm to 420 nm band has the strongest porphyrin photoexcitation coefficient.

However, blue light has poor depth of skin penetration.[5] Red light, however, in addition to its deeper penetration up to the sebaceous glands,[6] may have anti-inflammatory properties by influencing cytokine release from macrophages. According to an action spectrum for the inactivation of *P. acnes*, the sensitivity of *P. acnes* is highest for shorter wavelengths and decreases with increasing wavelength.

There are several studies showing the efficacy of blue light, and combination of both blue and red light for the treatment of mild to moderate acne (Table 16.2). The results uniformly showed short-term improvement in inflammatory lesions with blue light but none of the studies showed follow-up results beyond 12 weeks after treatment. Acne clearing is variable among patients and relapse rates are high after therapy is discontinued. One study out of two showed that combination of blue red light is superior to blue light alone.

PHOTODYNAMIC THERAPY (PDT)

It involves the application of ALA, which, when taken up by the pilosebaceous units, is metabolized through the heme synthesis pathway to produce protoporphyrin IX which when photoactivated, the resultant singlet oxygen and free radicals produced are cytotoxic resulting in the death of *P. acnes* and damage to the pilosebaceous unit itself.[7]

PDT requires 3 factors, a photosensitiser, light and oxygen. The commonly used photosensitizers are 5-aminolevulinic acid or, methyl aminolevulinate (MAL) and the newer ones are indocyanine green (ICG) and indole-3-acetic acid. Sources of light used are light emitting diodes, fluorescent lamps, IPL (filtered xenon flashlamps), filtered incandescent or arc lamps, lasers and sunlight. There are certain variables that influence *P. acnes* photoinactivation which include concentration of porphyrins (depending on type of acne lesion), effective fluence, wavelength of emitted photons, temperature at which the reaction is carried out and tissue oxygen availability.

Various studies have been conducted using PDT with ALA, MAL and ICG.[8] Most of the studies and their data are short-term and data is limited. However, the data shows that inflammatory lesions respond better to the various light sources of PDT in cases of mild to moderate acne.

COMPLICATIONS

In general, as lasers used for acne treatment are nonablative in nature, these treatments have little potential for significant complications. Most patients can expect erythema and edema lasting less than 24 hours.

LASERS IN MANAGEMENT OF ACNE SCARS

Lasers in particular have a central role in the management of acne scarring, which tends to be refractory to medical therapies.

The fractional lasers are predominantly used for the atrophic scars. The clinical implication of the depth of penetration of the lasers is particularly relevant in treating acne scars.

Acne scars are usually a mix of ice pick, boxcar and rolling scars, the final effect of fractional lasers largely depends on the predominant scars and the type of laser used.

For atrophic acne scars, it is important to choose a modality that reaches the appropriate depth to target the deep, boxcar and ice pick scars while concomitantly treating the superficial scars.

The rolling scars are a consequence of the destruction of the subcuticular fat, which leads to abnormal fibrous anchoring of the dermis to the subcutis.

Ice pick scars are narrow (<2 mm), deep, sharply marginated epithelial tracts that extend vertically to the deep dermis or subcutaneous tissue apex and it is believed that their depth is below than the depth of conventional skin resurfacing options and they rarely respond to fractional lasers.

Boxcar scars may be shallow (0.1–0.5 mm) or deep (0.5 mm) and are most often 1.5–4.0 mm in diameter. Logically, shallow boxcar scars and most deep boxcar scars are amenable to fractional lasers.

The depth–width ratio (DWR) for most fractional lasers is about 4–5 mm. The higher the DWR, more the dermal volume that can be thermally damaged. As the width of most fractional lasers is almost the same due to the intrinsic quality of the fractional 'technology', the depth is the variable factor that may play a predominant role in fractional laser efficacy.

REFERENCES

1. Cho SB, Lee SJ, Kang JM, Kim YK, Chung WS, Oh SH. The efficacy and safety of 10,600-nm carbon dioxide fractional laser for acne scars in Asian patients. Dermatologic Surgery. 2009 Dec;35(12):1955–61.
2. Manuskiatti W, Triwongwaranat D, Varothai S, Eimpunth S, Wanitphakdeedecha R. Efficacy and safety of a carbon-dioxide ablative fractional resurfacing device for treatment of atrophic acne scars in Asians. Journal of the American Academy of Dermatology. 2010 Aug 1;63(2):274–83.
3. Chapas AM, Brightman L, Sukal S, Hale E, Daniel D, Bernstein LJ, Geronemus RG. Successful treatment of acneiform scarring with CO_2 ablative fractional resurfacing. Lasers in Surgery and Medicine: The Official Journal of the American Society for Laser Medicine and Surgery. 2008 Aug;40(6):381–6.
4. Cameli N, Mariano M, Serio M, Ardigò M. Preliminary comparison of fractional laser with fractional laser plus radiofrequency for the treatment of acne scars and photoaging. Dermatologic Surgery. 2014 May;40(5):553–61.
5. Kjeldstad B. Different photoinactivation mechanisms in Propionibacterium acnes for near-ultraviolet and visible light. Photochem Photobiol 1987;46:363–6.
6. Elman M, Slatkine M, Harth Y. The effective treatment of acne vulgaris by a high-intensity, narrow band 405–420 nm light source. J Cosmet Laser Ther 2003;5:111–7.
7. Orfelt C, Stenquist B, Larko O, Faergemann J, Wennberg AM. Photodynamic therapy for acne vulgaris: A pilot study of the dose-response and mechanism of action. Acta Derm Venereol 2007;87:325–9.
8. Taub AF. Photodynamic therapy for the treatment of acne: A pilot study. J Drugs Dermatol 2004;3:S10–4.

CHAPTER

17

Cleansers, Moisturizers and Sunscreens in Acne

INTRODUCTION

Cleansing has evolved immensely over the years from simply scraping the skin to an exercise in relaxation and improvement in the skin's health and appearance. In disorders like acne, atopic dermatitis, rosacea, photoaging, 'sensitive skin', occupational dermatoses and also prior to aesthetic procedures, cleansing definitely has a beneficial role along with other therapeutic measures. However, a fine balance needs to be maintained between skin cleansing and the preservation of its homeostatic properties.[1]

MECHANISM

Substances capable of emulsifying the water insoluble environmental impurities and cosmetic products into finer particles are to be used for making these fat soluble impurities water soluble. Skin cleansers are surface-active substances (i.e. surfactants/soaps/emulsifiers/detergents) which reduce the surface tension on the skin and remove sebum, oil from cosmetic products, microorganisms, dirt and exfoliated cells. An ideal cleanser should do all these without causing damage or irritation and should keep the skin surface moist.[2]

Surfactants are the principal constituents of most cleansers. They move to the interface upon dissolving in water and lower the interfacial tension.[3] Surfactants can be ionic (anionic, cationic, amphoteric), nonionic, and silicone containing. Soap is the prototype anionic surfactant used in skin cleansers.

SOAPS

They are composed of long chain fatty acid alkali salts (pH of 9–10).

Syndet Bars

Synthetic detergents, when formulated into bar soaps, are known as 'syndets.' They offer the advantage of a neutral pH and are less likely to cause skin irritation and xerosis and do not form a soap scum layer. They have a non-soap synthetic surfactant as their principal ingredient. Transmission electron microscopy has shown that use of syndets leads to well-preserved lipid and protein regions compared to significant damage to both after washing with soap.[4]

Adverse Effects of Soaps

Harsh cleansers like soaps are known to cause:

1. Skin irritation
2. After wash tightness
3. Skin dryness, scaling and roughness
4. Allergic contact dermatitis

   Factors responsible for dryness and irritation in cleansers:

   i. **Surfactant ingredients:** Surfactants bind to keratin, causing protein denaturation and leading to cell membrane damage of keratinocytes resulting in adverse cutaneous responses.[5] Surfactant chain length is also an important factor in determining the irritant potential.[3]

   ii. **Skin cleanser residue or rinsability factor:** The irritancy potential of a cleansing agent may increase the longer it is left on the skin.

   iii. **pH of cleansing agent:** Soaps with an alkaline pH may cause damage to the lipid bilayer of the stratum corneum leading to dryness of the skin.[5] Although controversial, but still many dermatologist believe that maintaining the skin surface at its physiological pH (4–6.5) during cleansing prevents overgrowth of certain microorganisms, like *Propionibacterium acnes*.[6] However, some studies have shown that the pH of a cleanser plays a very little role in damaging the skin.[3]

It can be said that synthetic detergents and lipid-free cleansers have the least irritancy potential compared to other market products which have been proven in a recent study comparing various cleansers available in the Indian market.[7]

CLEANSING IN ACNE

The aim of cleansing in patients of acne or with acne-prone skin is to gently remove surface dirt, excessive skin lipids and sweat without causing dryness or irritation. The ideal cleanser for acne should be:

1. Noncomedogenic
2. Nonirritating
3. Nonallergenic[8]

It is a myth associated with acne that vigorous scrubbing of the skin with soap and water several times a day leads to reduced oiliness. However, this only results in aggravation of acne and it may even cause acne detergicans sometimes.

A large variety of skin cleansing agents is available for acne prone patients. This includes syndets, astringents, lipid free cleansers, abrasives and exfoliants.[9] The most common side effects of most antiacne therapies are dryness and irritation of the skin, hence it is important that gentle cleansing be done in these group of patients.

A liquid cleanser with good rinsability or a nonionic, fragrance-free dermatologic bar is the preferred choice in acne. The benefit of syndet cleansers specifically for acne patients has been demonstrated in studies in comparison to soaps.

Triclosan and Triclocarban are antimicrobials found in various cleansers including 'antibacterial soaps' marketed for acne management. In addition to having effects against *P. acnes*, these are also effective against Gram-positive bacteria and triclocarban is also effective against Gram- negative bacteria.

Many cleanser products contain fatty alcohols like cetyl alcohol, stearyl alcohol and cetearyl alcohol. These are typically derived from natural fats and oils. They can be wiped off without water. The fatty alcohols in these lotions facilitate evaporation and so rinsability is high. When used on the face, there is less facial residue which is an advantage of these lipid free-cleansing lotions.[6] These act as good emollients, emulsifiers and thickeners ultimately helping to moisturize the skin and countering the irritancy and drying potential. The cleansing regimen should be modified so that it suits the requirements of the individual patient.[8]

Soaps formulated specially for acne contain various ingredients such as sulfur, resorcinol, benzoyl peroxide or salicylic acid for their different beneficial effects on the acne prone skin.

Sulfur exhibits antimicrobial properties and has been in use medicinally since a long time. It is thought to be clinically effective in the treatment of acne partially due to its keratolytic effects because of the interaction between the keratinocyte and the cysteine component of sulfur. Sulfur is usually combined with other topical agents, such as benzoyl peroxide, salicylic acid and resorcinol.

Resorcinol is thought to have intrinsic keratolytic, antibacterial and antifungal activity but is believed to be ineffective as monotherapy. Both of these can cause mild irritation and sensitization. Also, there is associated malodor with sulfur products.

Benzoyl Peroxide Cleansers

As BPO is directly toxic to *P. acnes* and other bacteria, it has not been associated with the development of *P. acnes* resistance.[10–14] Studies with leave-on formulations of BPO demonstrate reduction in the emergence of antibiotic-resistant *P. acnes* strains in patients treated concurrently with topical antibiotics, such as erythromycin or clindamycin.[10–14]

A BPO cleanser/wash is designed to be used during the process of washing the skin followed by rinsing. Data regarding the microbiologic effects and efficacy of available BPO cleanser/wash formulations are limited.[15, 16]

However, a few studies using BPO wash/cleanser have revealed modest to marked reduction of *P. acnes*, marked reduction of the colony counts of *P. acnes* strains shown prior to treatment to be resistant to one or more antibiotics and also shown its effectiveness in the treatment of acne vulgaris.[16–21]

Cleanser use may be better tolerated due to leave-on side effects of BP such as irritation and bleaching of clothes.[6]

Alfa-hydroxy Acids

These are water soluble, penetrate the epidermis and even into the dermis at higher concentrations. The mechanism of action is desquamation of stratum corneum (exfoliation). Specifically, they disrupt corneocyte adhesion in the upper stratum corneum, possibly by chelating calcium. These also promote epidermolysis, disperse basal layer melanin and may increase collagen synthesis if they are strong enough to penetrate the dermis.[22] This leads to a smoother appearance of the skin clinically, and may make them helpful for acne prevention and treatment of post-inflammatory hyperpigmentation. Examples include glycolic, lactic and citric acid.

Beta-hydroxy Acids

The only beta-hydroxy acid used in dermatology is salicylic acid. It is lipid-soluble allowing it to penetrate not only the epidermis but also the pilosebaceous unit. This makes it comedolytic, resulting in its superiority over alfa-hydroxy acids in treating acne. It also has an anti-inflammatory action. There are various studies demonstrating the superiority of salicylic acid to placebo or to benzoyl peroxide.[23]

Poly-hydroxy Acids

These have been shown to be less irritating than alfa-hydroxy acids and include lactobionic acid and gluconolactone. These have a slower and gentler absorption rate and are compatible for clinically sensitive skin.[24]

SCRUBS

When it was observed that desquamation of the stratum corneum can lead to younger and smoother-appearing skin, abrasive scrubs were developed. These may contain different types of abrasives like aluminum oxide and ground fruit pits (most common), polyethylene beads or sodium tetraborate decahydrate granules (least abrasive).[25] It is believed that abrasion unroofs the closed comedones and prevents their progression.[26] However, this may lead to irritant effects by damaging the functional integrity of the stratum corneum, augmenting the potential for cutaneous irritation with other topical acne therapies. Hence these are not recommended for patients with sensitive skin.

MOISTURIZERS

Recent evidence has shown that acne by itself and certain medications prescribed for its treatment may cause dysfunction of epidermal barrier with increase in trans-epidermal water loss (TEWL) and lead to symptoms of dryness, redness, subjective irritation, pruritus, increased skin sensitivity and discomfort to the patient. This can lead to nonadherence with treatment and treatment failure focuses on four primary fundamental goals:

1. Cleansing
2. Medicating
3. Moisturizing, and
4. Photoprotection.[27]

Causes of Epidermal Barrier Dysfunction in Acne Vulgaris

Epidermal barrier impairment innate to acne vulgaris: Patients with acne vulgaris had markedly diminished levels of free sphingosine, linoleic acid and total ceramides in stratum corneum, causing deficiency of the intercellular lipid membrane, leading to increased TEWL (Trans-epidermal water loss) and stratum corneum permeability barrier dysfunction.[28] It is hypothesized that ceramide deficiency resulting in impaired skin barrier can promote follicular hyperkeratosis leading to comedone formation.

Medication-induced epidermal changes:

Benzoyl peroxide: Benzoyl peroxide has been shown to adversely affect the epidermal barrier function by causing impairment in the antioxidant barrier and stratum corneum permeability barrier.[29]

Retinoids: Retinoids (both oral and topical) cause accelerated epidermal cell turnover with thickening of lower epidermis and thinning of stratum corneum with micro-fissure formation. This together with an increased TEWL leads to compromised stratum corneum barrier function. This manifests as "retinoid dermatitis" characterized by erythema, fine scaling, desquamation and irritation, which usually happens within the initial 1–3 weeks of therapy. It was observed that use of moisturizer 2 weeks prior and during tretinoin treatment prevented an increase in TEWL and improved symptoms of retinoid dermatitis.[30]

Patients having acne with other skin conditions: Moisturizers may also need to be prescribed in individuals with acne who have co-existent atopic dermatitis, sensitive skin or are living in climatic conditions with severe winters or low humidity as all these can cause impairment of the epidermal barrier and associated skin sensitivity.

Constituents of Various Moisturizers Used for Acne (Fig. 17.1)

An ideal moisturizer should be non-comedogenic and should not worsen acne, should have no sensitization or irritation potential, diminish facial shine and skin oiliness, decrease the TEWL,

Table 17.1: Ingredients of moisturizers for acne

Properties	*Ingredients*
Occlusive	Beeswax, caprylic/capric triglyceride, cetyl alcohol, cocoa butter, cyclomethicone, dimethicone, glyceryl stearate, grape seed oil, lanolin (wool alcohol), lecithin
Humectant	Betaine, butylene glycol, cetearyl isononanoate, glycerin (glycerol), honey, hyaluronic acid, jojoba oil, lactic acid
Emollient	Almond oil, arachidyl alcohol, cetearyl alcohol, cholesterol, cyclomethicone, cyclopentasiloxane, decyl oleate, dimethicone, ethylhexyl palmitate, fatty acids, glyceryl stearate, isohexadecane, isopropyl myristate, lanolin (wool alcohol)
Anti-inflammatory	Aloe vera (Aloe barbadensis), beeswax, bisabolol, chamomile (*Matricaria recutita*), coconut oil, cucumber extract, glycyrrhetinic acid, green tea extract, *Hypericum perforatum* (St. John's wort), licochalcone A, benzoyl peroxide
Oil reducing	Licochalcone A

increase the skin hydration, should be cosmetically acceptable and incorporate a broad-spectrum photoprotection. In a study by Chularojanamontri et al. 52 products of moisturizers that are available online and over-the-counter and which claim to be suitable for acne were selected and their ingredients and properties were identified.[31]

SUNSCREENS

Sun exposure in acne patients has a big impact on the progression of the disease, because it can promote bacterial proliferation and reduce immune response, thus favoring inflammation (Fig. 17.1). Therefore, it is essential to explain the importance of sun protection to the patient. In this regard, light and non-occlusive products, in the form of sprays, gels or liquids, should be preferred. UVA and UVB rays affect acne differently. UVA rays, specifically UVA1 and blue light (400 nm) may have anti-inflammatory effects. In contrast, UVB

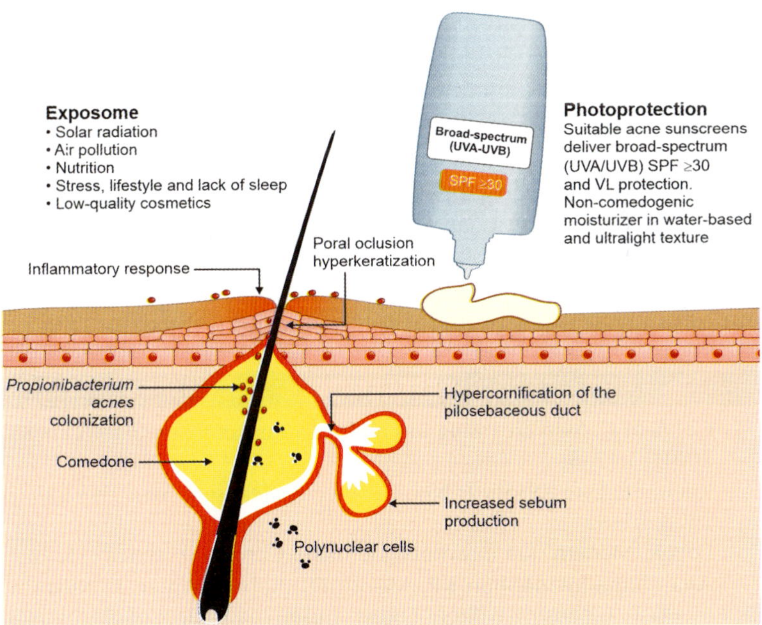

Fig. 17.1: Sunlight in the pathogenesis of acne[33]

Table 17.2: Ingredient of sunscreen and it's properties

Ingredient	*Non-comedogenic qualities*	*Potential for irritation*
Zinc oxide	Excellent	Minimal
Titanium dioxide	Excellent	Minimal
Iron oxide	Good	Low
Silica	Good	Low
Octinoxate	Poor	High
Octisalate	Poor	Moderate
Avobenzone	Poor	Moderate to high

rays cause inflammation, and increase sebum production and proliferation of keratinocytes.[32,33]

Retinoids not only stimulate desquamation and melanocyte disbursal, but they also directly affect pigmentation by blocking melanosome transfer to the keratinocyte while increasing epidermal turnover. Moreover, irritation due to retinoid use may potentially worsen post-inflammatory hyperpigmentation (PIH). Therefore, regular sunscreen use is recommended to minimize retinoid-induced photodermatitis.[34] Other oral photosensitizing drugs are the tetracyclines. Ideal sunscreen should be non-comedogenic. Zinc oxide and titanium dioxide are preferred (Table 17.2).

A prospective open-label study ($n = 91$) of acne patients under treatment with diverse acne medications (oral and/or topical) showed that the daily use of a cleanser plus a sunscreen SPF30 with emollient properties improved skin tolerability, helped patients to not miss applications of therapies, and could reduce the TEWL.[35]

REFERENCES

1. Gelmetti C. Skin cleansing in children. J EurAcad Dermatol Venereol 2001;15:12–5.
2. Kuehl BL, Fyfe KS, Shear NH. Cutaneous cleansers. Skin Therapy Lett 2003;8:1–4.
3. Ertel K. Modern skin cleansers. Dermatol Clin 2000;18:561–75.
4. Ananthapadmanabhan KP, Moore DJ, Subramanyan K, Misra M, Meyer F. Cleansing without compromise: The impact of cleansers on the skin barrier and the technology of mild cleansing. Dermatol Ther 2004;17:16–25.

5. Bikowski J. The use of cleansers as therapeutic concomitants in various dermatologic disorders. Cutis 2001;68:12–9.
6. Stringer T, Nagler A, Orlow SJ, Oza VS. Clinical evidence for washing and cleansers in acne vulgaris: a systematic review. Journal of Dermatological Treatment. 2018 Oct 3;29(7):688–93.
7. Lakshmi C, Srinivas CR, Anand CV, Mathew AC. Irritancy ranking of 31 cleansers in the Indian market in a 24-h patch test. Int J Cosmet Sci 2008;30:277–83.
8. Solomon BA, Shalita AR. Effect of detergents in acne. Clin Dermatol 1996;14:95–9.
9. Toombs EL. Cosmetics in treatment of acne vulgaris. Dermatol Clin 2005;23:575–81.
10. Gollnick H, Cunliffe W, Berson D, et al. Management of acne: a report from a global alliance to improve outcomes in acne. J Am Acad Dermatol. 2003;49:S1–S37.
11. Leyden JJ, Del Rosso JQ, Webster GF. Clinical considerations in the treatment of acne vulgaris and other inflammatory skin disorders: focus on antibiotic resistance. Cutis. 2007;79(6 Suppl):9–25.
12. Tanghetti EA, Papp KF. A current review of topical benzoyl peroxide: new perspectives on formulation and utilization. Dermatol Clin. 2009.
13. Cunliffe WJ, Holland KT, Bojar R, et al.A randomized, double-blind comparison of a clindamycin phosphate/ benzoyl peroxide gel formulation and a matching clindamycin gel with respect to microbiologic activity and clinical efficacy in the topical treatment of acne vulgaris. Clin Ther. 2002;24:1117–1133.
14. Del Rosso JQ, Leyden JJ, Thiboutot D, et al. Antibiotic use in cane vulgaris and rosacea: clinical considerations and resistance issues of significance to dermatologists. Cutis. 2008;82 (Suppl 2S[ii]):5–12.
15. Del Rosso JQ. Benzoyl peroxide cleanser formulations for treatment of acne vulgaris: status report on available data. Cutis. 2008.
16. Del Rosso JQ. Therapeutic cleansers. Skin & Aging. 2003 (Aug):80–85.
17. Mills OH, Rafal E, Hino P, et al. Data on file. Fort Worth, TX: Galderma Laboratories; 2002. Evaluating the efficacy of benzoyl peroxide wash.
18. Leyden JJ, Kaidbey K. Data on file. Scottsdale, AZ: Medicis Pharmaceuticals; 2002. Evaluation of the antimicrobial effects in vivo of benzoyl peroxide cleanser (Triaz) in humans.
19. Leyden JJ. The effect of benzoyl peroxide 6% wash on antibiotic-resistant Propionibacterium acnes. Poster presented at: 31st Hawaii Dermatology Seminar; March 3–9, 2007; Wailea, Maui, Hawaii.
20. Shalita AR, Rafal ES, Anderson D, et al. Compared efficacy and safety of tretinoin 0.1% microsphere gel alone and in combination with benzoyl peroxide 6% cleanser for the treatment of cane vulgaris. Cutis. 2003;72:167–72.

21. Gold M. Survey results of compliance, preference, and satisfaction in patients prescribed benzoyl peroxide 8% wash and benzoyl peroxide 9% cleanser for the treatment of acne vulgaris. Poster presented at: American Academy of Dermatology Annual Meeting; March 2006; San Francisco, California.
22. Tung RC, Bergfeld WF, Vidimos AT, Remzi BK. Alpha hydroxy acid based cosmetic procedures: guidelines for patient management. Am J Clin Dermatol. 2000;1(2):81–8.
23. Shalita, A. R. "Comparison of a salicylic acid cleanser and a benzoyl peroxide wash in the treatment of acne vulgaris." Clinical therapeutics 11.2 (1988): 264–7.
24. Grimes PE, Green BA, Wildnauer RH, et al. The use of polyhydroxy acids (PHAs) in photoaged skin. Cutis. 2004;73 (Suppl 2):3–13.
25. Draelos ZD. Reexamining methods of facial cleansing. Cosmetic Dermatol. 2005;18(2):173–5.
26. Mills OH, Kligman AM. Evaluation of abrasives in acne therapy. Cutis. 1979;23(5):704–5.
27. Stringer T, Nagler A, Orlow SJ, Oza VS. Clinical evidence for washing and cleansers in acne vulgaris: a systematic review. Journal of Dermatological Treatment. 2018 Oct 3;29(7):688–93.
28. Del Rosso JQ, Gold M, Rueda MJ, Brandt S, Winkelman WJ. Efficacy, safety, and subject satisfaction of a specified skin care regimen to cleanse, medicate, moisturize, and protect the skin of patients under treatment for acne vulgaris. The Journal of Clinical and Aesthetic Dermatology. 2015 Jan;8(1):22.
29. Thiboutot D, Del Rosso JQ. Acne vulgaris and the epidermal barrier: is acne vulgaris associated with inherent epidermal abnormalities that cause impairment of barrier functions? Do any topical acne therapies alter the structural and/or functional integrity of the epidermal barrier?. The Journal of Clinical and Aesthetic Dermatology. 2013 Feb;6(2):18.
30. Yamamoto A, Takenouchi K, Ito M. Impaired water barrier function in acne vulgaris. Archives of Dermatological Research. 1995 Feb; 287:214–8.
31. Chularojanamontri L, Tuchinda P, Kulthanan K, Pongparit K. Moisturizers for acne: What are their constituents? The Journal of clinical and aesthetic dermatology. 2014 May;7(5):36.
32. Conforti C, Giuffrida R, Fadda S, Fai A, Romita P, Zalaudek I, Dianzani C. Topical dermocosmetics and acne vulgaris. Dermatologic Therapy. 2021 Jan;34(1):e14436.
33. Piquero-Casals J, Morgado-Carrasco D, Rozas-Muñoz E, Mir-Bonafé JF, Trullàs C, Jourdan E, Piquero-Martin J, Zouboulis CC, Krutmann J. Sun exposure, a relevant exposome factor in acne patients and how photoprotection can improve outcomes. Journal of Cosmetic Dermatology. 2023 Jun;22(6):1919–28.

34. How KN, Ho WC, Sundaran M, Wan Ahmal Kammal WS, Lim PY, Chew W. Efficacy and Tolerability of a Sunscreen Containing Licochalcone A and L-Carnitine as an Adjunct to Retinoids in the Management of Acne and Post-Acne Pigmentation Among Malaysian Patients. Clinical, Cosmetic and Investigational Dermatology. 2023 Dec 31:3719–29.
35. Del Rosso JQ, Brandt S. The role of skin care as an integral component in the management of acne vulgaris: part 2: tolerability and performance of a designated skin care regimen using a foam wash and moisturizer SPF 30 in patients with acne vulgaris undergoing active treatment. The Journal of Clinical and Aesthetic Dermatology. 2013 Dec;6(12):28.

Index